London: New Holland, 2006   1845370309

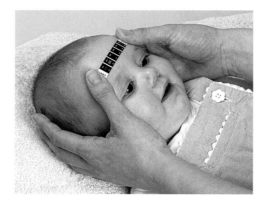

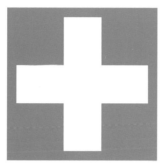

FIRST
AID
for
Babies
& Children

First published in 2006 by New Holland Publishers Ltd.
London • Cape Town • Sydney • Auckland
• 86 Edgware Road, London W2 2EA, United Kingdom
• 80 McKenzie Street, Cape Town 8001, South Africa
• 14 Aquatic Drive, Frenchs Forest NSW 2086, Australia
• 218 Lake Road, Northcote, Auckland, New Zealand

www.newhollandpublishers.com

ISBN (HB)   1 84537 030 9
ISBN (PB)   1 84537 031 7

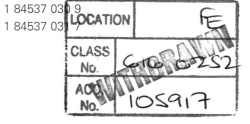

The Publishers wish to thank the models for participating in
the various photoshoots: Ulla and Amber Bothe; Amy Chaplin;
Emma Charles; Lexie and Gina du Toit; Ashleigh Hamilton;
Catherine, Georgia, Joshua and Denim Haywood; Noah
Innes; Jamie Knowles; Shirley, Hannah, Joshua and David
Lim; Tyler Miller; Kerry and Brenna Nel; Debra and Savannah
Orffer-Brown; Benjamin and Claire Rideout; Thomas, Lilly
and Ella Waterkeyn; Claudia and Elvano Willemse.

Publishing Managers: Claudia Dos Santos and Simon Pooley
Commissioning Editor: Alfred LeMaitre
Editors: Di Kilpert and Roxanne Reid
Designer: Lyndall du Toit
Photographers: Lisa Trocchi, Isabel Koorts and Luke Calder
Illustrator: Ian Lusted
Picture Researcher: Karla Kik
Production: Myrna Collins
Proofreader/indexer: Sylvia Grobbelaar

Reproduction by Resolution Colour (Pty) Ltd., Cape Town, SA
Printed and bound in Malaysia by Times Offset (M) Sdn. Bhd.

10 9 8 7 6 5 4 3 2 1

The life-support techniques and sequences in this book are
modelled on those devised and advocated by the Advanced
Life Support Group (ALSG) in the United Kingdom. They
have been used extensively for the training of healthcare
professionals in Europe, South Africa and Australia.

DISCLAIMER

Although the author and publisher have made every effort to ensure
that the information contained in this book was accurate at the time
of going to press, they accept no responsbility for any loss, injury or
inconvenience sustained by any person using this book or following
the advice given in it.

PICTURE CREDITS

Mediscan p52; Prof. Heather Zar p110 bottom; Science Photo
pp10, 112 top, 116 top right, 130, 132–134, 135 right, 136 top and
middle right, 137 top, 138 bottom right, 139, 140.

FOREWORD

'My mother had a great deal of trouble with me, but I think she enjoyed it.'
Mark Twain

The joy of seeing children grow and develop is inevitably marred on occasion by minor mishaps and illnesses, which cause the parent or care-giver considerable anxiety. A health professional is not often on the spot at such times, and it is up to you to cope. This book will not give a detailed account of injuries and medical conditions that affect children. It is intended to help you manage the injury or illness yourself in an emergency, and will give guidance on whether and when further professional help is needed. Such help varies greatly according to circumstances. It might be a general practitioner who knows the whole family well, a paediatrician, or a nurse. It might be a clinic down the road, or a health centre many miles away. Guidance will also be given as to how soon such help is needed – next week will do, or should it be tomorrow? An emergency call for an ambulance, or a rushed journey to hospital by car will occasionally be required, and these unpleasant situations are described. Stick a list of important phone numbers at the back of this book – your doctor, an ambulance service, the local hospital, the police. And make sure the book is readily available!

Prevention is the name of the game! A lot of discomfort, worry and money can be saved by preventing the problem in the first place. So space has been allocated to the important fields of injury prevention in and outside the home. Immunization is one of the most cost-effective measures we have to prevent certain illnesses – not only in your own child but in the community at large. There are many misconceptions about immunization, and you will find answers to commonly asked questions on this subject on pages 142–144.

CONTENTS

Part one

FIRST AID & HOME SAFETY

Part two

FIRST AID FOR MEDICAL CONDITIONS

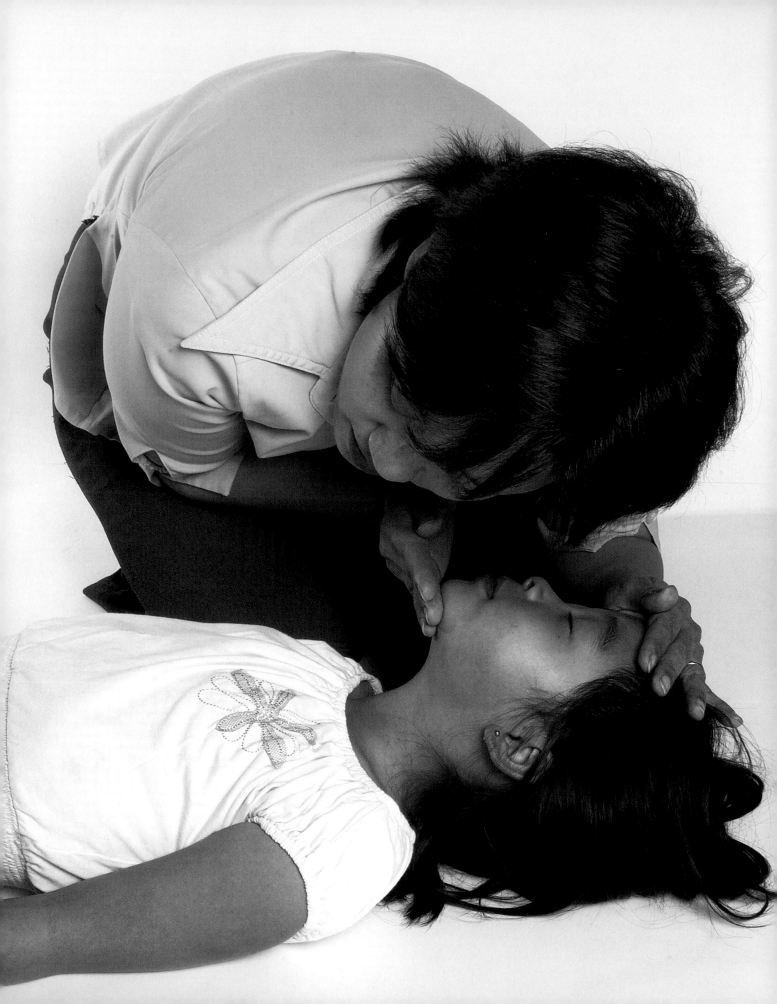

Part 1

First Aid & Home Safety

COPING IN AN EMERGENCY

We all hope that we will never be called upon to assist in a situation requiring us to provide first aid, but by preparing yourself beforehand you will know what to do. A knowledge of basic first-aid procedures will help you to be calm and efficient. The individual procedures in this book offer a range of specific instructions, but be sure to learn the basics at least and attend a recognized first-aid course.

In an emergency situation, a desire to provide meaningful care and comfort can easily dissolve into blind panic unless you have certain basic skills and a systematic approach to resuscitation procedures. This is well within anyone's capabilities! A little knowledge, insight and hands-on training in basic first aid will give you confidence in yourself. You will be amazed at how useful – and even heroic – you can be when the occasion demands.

This manual is not designed to turn you into an expert. What we offer you is a set of skills any responsible person can apply in a wide variety of emergencies involving children. In many respects, your role in a medical emergency may be the most vital of all. As a parent, guardian or child minder you are likely to be the first person on the scene when a child is injured or suddenly becomes ill. Equipped with the basic tools and practical skills covered in this book, you should be in a position to do your bit as the first responder, and perhaps avoid a visit to the local doctor or the hospital.

You may even save a life by applying basic life-support measures to a choking or unconscious child.

Once you have read the guidelines provided in this book you should go one step further and become a fully-fledged life-support provider. We recommend that you register for a lay person's course available in your area, which is endorsed by the national council or first aid service operating in your country. Most recognized courses will not only teach you valuable life-support sequences designed to deal with almost any medical emergency, but will allow you to practise and fine-tune your skills on lifelike manikins.

Note:
To simplify, we refer to the 'child' (aged one to eight years) throughout this book, though of course infants (under one year of age) are included. If treatments or first-aid procedures differ for an infant this is specified.

Please remember

Not only is prevention always better than cure – it can also save your child pain and you much heartache. We sincerely believe that almost every injury can be prevented, and you should believe this too. For that reason we have included some practical hints and measures aimed at reducing the risk of accidents in and around the home (*see* pages 31–37). Putting these simple measures into practice will cost you time, effort and perhaps even money, but just consider the alternative. Do you really want to tempt risk, fate or disaster? Of course not!

ROLE OF THE FIRST RESPONDER

Most serious injuries and medical emergencies occur without warning. Trained medical personnel may not be able to get to the scene of an accident in time and so the outcome – sometimes the difference between life and death – often depends on just two factors:
• how quickly basic life support is provided

- whether anyone at the scene can assess nature and severity of the situation, call for appropriate assistance and, if necessary, commence resuscitation procedures (*see* pages 18-21) until help arrives.

Particularly in life-threatening emergencies such as near drowning (*see* pages 96-99), choking (*see* pages 28-30) and severe bleeding (*see* page 9), survival often depends upon whether the first responder can initiate effective resuscitation while waiting for help. As a parent, grandparent, teacher, child-minder or sports coach you should have the skills necessary to take decisive action.

Call for help

Call for assistance before you commence first aid if the infant or child is:

- unconscious, drowsy or disoriented
- having difficulty breathing or is not breathing at all
- suffering from multiple injuries, or burns
- bleeding heavily from one or more wounds
- suspected of having ingested a poisonous substance.

If you are unsure of the cause of the collapse or injury, another reliable person should phone for assistance while you commence first aid. If you are alone, phone for help first before you start resuscitation procedures. Whom you call depends on the services that are available in your area.

What to say on the phone:
Calm down and speak clearly so that you do not have to repeat yourself unnecessarily. You must provide basic information:

- your **name and contact telephone number**
- your **location** (physical address), and possibly directions as well
- a brief **description of the incident**

Do not hang up until you are told to do so. The dispatcher may be able to give you helpful assistance.

EMERGENCY NUMBERS

Keep a record of emergency contacts next to your telephone, in your diary and in the directory of your mobile phone. *See* page 157 for an emergency list. Also inform your children – even toddlers can memorize their home address and the (usually simple) numbers to dial for emergency response.

Assess the injured child

Temper your enthusiasm with good judgement: look before you leap in, regardless of the seeming severity of the emergency. Any situation you encounter should be calmly and objectively assessed before you decide on your best course of action.

Protect yourself and the injured child from further danger

In a potentially dangerous environment, good judgement is essential to ensure everyone's safety including your own. Even if you are the only one who is able to provide help you must never put your own life at risk.

Giving first aid

If a child is unconscious, in shock, or breathing with difficulty, the speed with which you restore normal breathing and blood circulation is the single most important factor. In many instances, the care required from you as first responder may be fairly straightforward; no outside help may be necessary. At other times the extent and severity of the condition may not be clearly apparent and your quick response will give the casualty the best possible chance of recovery.

FIRST-AID KITS

You should always have a first-aid kit handy in your home and vehicle, and whenever you engage in outdoor pursuits, such as hiking or camping with your children. Many commerically available ready-made kits suit the most basic of needs, but consider making your own one or supplementing a bought kit, so that it takes into account the ages and specific requirements of your family members.

Check on expiry dates from time to time to ensure that your supply is not out of date and ensure that all first-aid kits and their contents are safe from small, enquiring hands and stored in a safe, lockable place.

Putting a kit together

If you decide to design your own first-aid kit, choose a container that is durable, preferably waterproof, and big enough to contain all the items so that you can see and get at them easily without having to tip them all out. Carry-alls for fishing tackle, or small toolboxes are ideal because they have convenient compartments.

On the lid of your first-aid kit, stick a list of useful telephone numbers (*see* page 157) – such as your family doctor, local clinic or hospital, poison centre, ambulance service, next-door neighbour and neighbourhood security patrol.

When you decide what to include, do not overstock. Simply remember to replace whatever you use, and check the kit at least once a year to ensure that nothing is lacking to cater for the changing needs of your growing children.

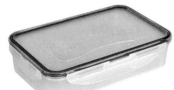

An inexpensive plastic lunchbox makes an ideal container for a small basic first-aid kit.

Your first-aid shopping list

- One sturdy container

Instruments

- 1 small pair of sharp stainless steel scissors
- 1 large pair of dressmaker's scissors, for cutting bandages and plasters
- 1 pair of fine tweezers for removing dirt, thorns and other foreign bodies
- A few 19–21 gauge sterile injection needles for teasing out splinters
- A few sterile 5ml (1 teaspoon) syringes or measuring spoons, for giving oral medication to infants and toddlers
- An oral mercury thermometer or temperature strips (*see* Fever, page 103)
- A few paperclips, for draining blood from under nails
- A couple of large safety pins for keeping slings in place
- Two pairs of disposable surgical gloves
- Two small eye droppers

LATEX ALLERGY

Approximately 1% of adults may be allergic to gloves made from natural rubber latex. They usually get skin rashes or symptoms similar to hay fever, and sometimes wheezing and other severe reactions. You may be sensitive to latex if you are allergic to kiwi fruit, tomato, avocado, bananas or water chestnuts. If you think you may be at risk of latex allergy, rather use gloves made from synthetic latex or vinyl.

FIRST-AID KIT

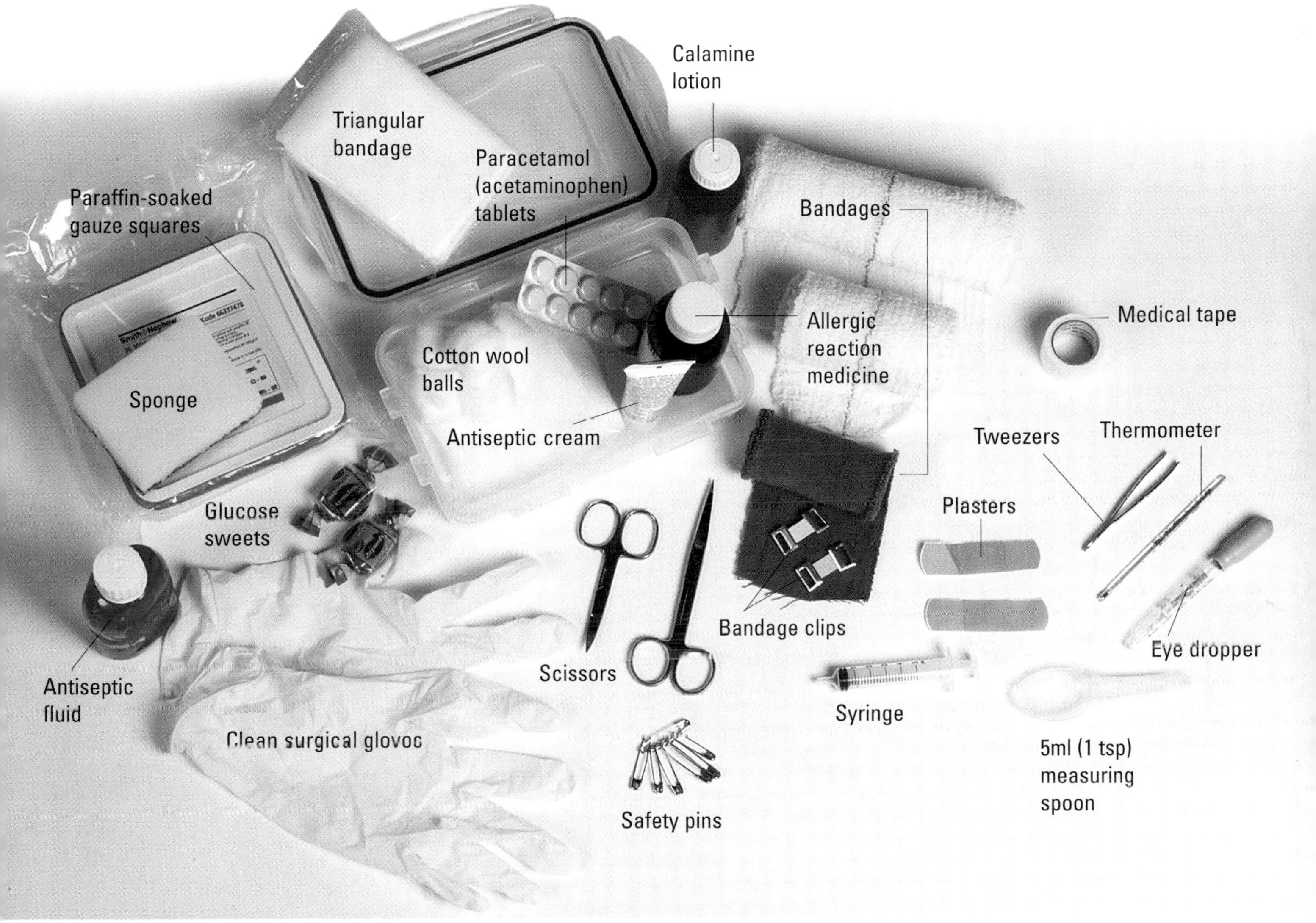

Calamine lotion

Triangular bandage

Paracetamol (acetaminophen) tablets

Paraffin-soaked gauze squares

Bandages

Sponge

Medical tape

Allergic reaction medicine

Cotton wool balls

Antiseptic cream

Tweezers

Thermometer

Glucose sweets

Plasters

Bandage clips

Antiseptic fluid

Eye dropper

Scissors

Clean surgical gloves

Syringe

5ml (1 tsp) measuring spoon

Safety pins

Oral medications
- Paracetamol (acetaminophen) in liquid or chewable tablet form for pain relief (do not give aspirin or anti-inflammatory medication to children under 12 years of age)
- Promethazine hydrochloride in syrup or tablet form for mild allergic reactions
- Glucose water or sweets

Topical medications
- Antiseptic solution (chlorhexidine) for cleaning wounds and instruments
- Povidone-iodine ointment for dressing wounds
- Calamine lotion for sunburn, rashes and minor skin irritations
- Cream or gel containing the local anaesthetic benzocaine, for insect bites and stings

Dressings

- 2 packs of sterile cotton wool balls or swabs
- 2 packs of sterile gauze pads
- 2 small dishwashing sponges for cleaning wounds
- 1 roll of hypoallergenic medical tape for securing dressings
- Gauze bandages – 2cm and 5cm width (³/₄in and 2in)
- Elastic bandages with clips
- Adhesive tape and bandages – 2.5cm and 5cm width (1in and 2in)

- 1 tin of paraffin-impregnated gauze squares
- Cotton sheeting and 1m (3ft) flannel strips for slings
- 2 eye protectors, made by cutting the bottom half off two polystyrene cups (*see* Eye Injuries, page 57)

To keep in your freezer

- A bag of frozen peas to use as a cold compress (*see* Bumps and Bruises, page 38)

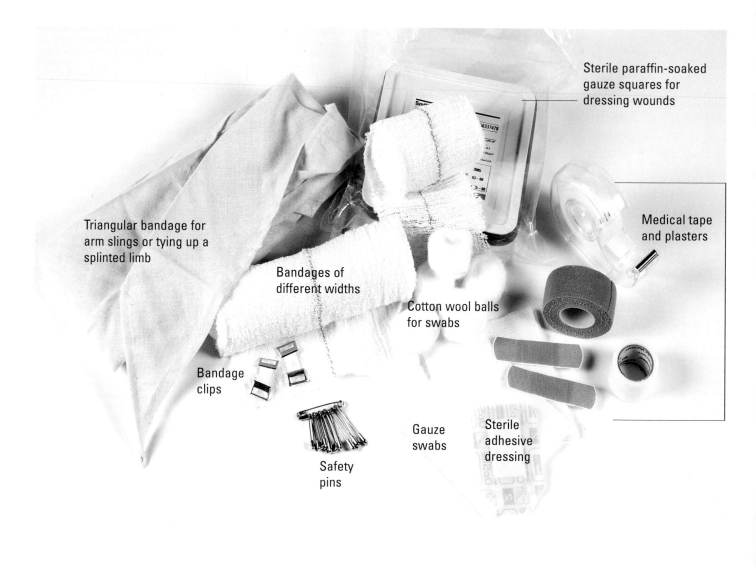

Sterile paraffin-soaked gauze squares for dressing wounds

Triangular bandage for arm slings or tying up a splinted limb

Bandages of different widths

Cotton wool balls for swabs

Medical tape and plasters

Bandage clips

Safety pins

Gauze swabs

Sterile adhesive dressing

Additional items for travel

- Sunscreen with a sufficiently high SPF
- Insect repellent
- Medicines prescribed and taken for chronic conditions (insulin, bronchodilators, and so on)
- Blankets for conserving warmth, particularly in cold weather
- Paper and pen or pencil for taking down telephonic instructions from the doctor

Some important tips

Accidents can happen next door or at the local playground and you may need to grab your kit and do a 'housecall'. So, even if you already have some of the listed items in your medicine cupboard, it is worth having duplicates in your first-aid kit as well.

Clean all non-disposable instruments with detergent and water after use, and dry them well (so they will not rust) before putting them back in the first-aid kit.

Use medicines only in the prescribed doses; check with your family doctor or local clinic that they are safe for your child.

Store your kit in a cool place, away from direct sunlight, and where it is out of the reach of small children but easily accessible to adults.

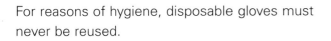

For reasons of hygiene, disposable gloves must never be reused.

STANDARD PRECAUTIONS

If you have completed a recognized basic first-aid course, and are ready to volunteer your skills in a medical emergency, always carry a few pairs of light surgical gloves around with you (*see* Latex Allergy, page 10). The main purpose of the gloves is to protect you from infection, so they need not be sterile, just clean and unbroken. Particularly if the person you are resuscitating is a stranger, always consider the possibility of communicable infectious diseases. This is especially important if you risk coming into contact with the subject's blood or other body fluids, for example:

- when performing mouth-to-mouth resuscitation, or if the person is bleeding from any site;
- you have a fresh skin wound of any size on your own hands or face;
- you live in a country or region where there is a high prevalence of infectious hepatitis or human immunodeficiency virus (HIV).

If you are obliged to administer life support without gloves, and even if it appears to your naked eye that no contamination with body fluids has occurred, always wash your hands thoroughly with soap and water as soon as possible afterward.

ACCIDENTS HAPPEN

There is nothing worse for a parent, teacher, grandparent, or caregiver than to see a child injured and in pain, or, worse yet, in dire need of medical attention. Children are adventurous and enthusiastic in their explorations of the world around them, and accidents are bound to happen some time. Luckily, serious mishaps are relatively rare, but it helps to be prepared in any case of emergency.

If you are first to arrive on the scene of a serious injury, you need to be able to take charge and direct additional helpers until medical support arrives. To be effective you must remain calm, and concentrate on what you have to do. The sooner effective treatment can begin, the better the potential for a positive outcome. The most urgent situation occurs when breathing ceases and the heart stops beating. This emergency takes precedence over anything else – any other injury.

WHAT YOU CAN DO TO HELP

Time is critical, so remain focused and follow the guidelines given below. Details of the rescue breathing procedure can be found on pages 18–27.

Determine the priorities
- Check the child's level of responsiveness (*see* Are you alright? on this page).
- As soon as possible check the child's airway and breathing (*see* pages 18–20).

- If the child is unconscious but breathing, place her in the recovery position (*see* page 23). Unconscious infants should be held in the recovery position as shown on page 26.
- Check if there is any visible bleeding; control the bleeding by applying pressure on the wound.

Are you alright? (*See also* page 17)
A child lying motionless on the ground may not be unconscious. However, if she does **not** respond to you, establish whether she is conscious and breathing.

Children between one and seven years old
Squeeze the child's hand, call her name if you know it, ask 'Are you alright?' or give a command such as 'Open your eyes!' If the child responds and speaks to you it indicates that the airway is clear and that the child is able to breathe – she is not unconscious.

If the child is drowsy, move her into the recovery position and stay with her until the emergency service arrives. A child who is in shock, or is bleeding, may be covered with a blanket to conserve body heat. If the child does not respond to you, call for help, open the airway and begin rescue breathing (*see* page 19).

Infants under one year old
Place the infant on his back directly in front of you, on a firm surface. Tap the sole of his foot and call his name. If the infant responds take him with you while you telephone for medical assistance.

If the infant fails to respond open his airway and begin rescue breathing (*see* page 27).

Monitor the child's responsiveness
An injured child may progress from being conscious to unconsciousness, her condition either improving or deteriorating fairly rapidly. A fully conscious child will be able to respond to your questions anything less is a cause for concern.

Watch out for the following signs which indicate depressed consciousness in a child:
- drowsy or difficult to arouse
- clearly disoriented (not able to tell you their name, which day it is, or where they are)
- slurred speech
- unable to answer easy questions correctly.

MOVING AN INJURED CHILD

As a general rule, resuscitation and first aid should be administered right where you have found the child, to ensure the quickest possible restoration of vital functions and reduce the serious risk of complications such as shock and the aggravation of injuries. While you commence first aid procedures on the spot, another reliable and responsible person should be sent to call for medical assistance immediately.

Severe injuries

Due to the risk of aggravating a possible spinal injury a seriously injured child should not be moved, though there are exceptions to this rule (*see* SAFE approach on page 16). Neck and spine injuries are very difficult to detect during a routine first-aid assessment, and any attempts to move someone with an injured spine can convert the condition from a relatively harmless to disastrous. It is advisable always to assume spinal injury in the following cases:
- an unconscious child
- obvious signs of a head injury
- sporting injuries (as a result of playing a contact sport, or a fall from a horse)
- in a child who complains of a painful neck or back
- if a child is unable to move arms or legs.

If you have reason to suspect a neck or spinal injury, ensure that the child lies still on a flat surface and that its head and neck are aligned (not bent forwards, backwards or sidewise, but kept in a neutral position).

Immobilize the neck with whatever you have to hand. Some stiffly rolled up towels or T-shirts can serve as handy subsitutes to prevent movement. Ensure that you stabilize the sides of the head and neck only – the throat must not be obstructed in any way, to prevent depressing the child's airway.

Exceptions to the rule
No matter what the injury, you must move a casualty to safety if:
- it is near a fire (*see* pages 72–76)
- it is in water (*see* pages 96–99)
- there is a toxic substance or gas nearby.

Minor injuries

Once first aid has been provided, a child with a minor injury can safely be moved to a more convenient or sheltered location. Bear in mind that fainting is quite common when an injured person (who has been lying on the ground) suddenly gets up. This is due a combination of factors such as emotional shock, pain and minor blood loss. It is best to stay with the child and guide its steps as it walks.

Injury in remote places

In a remote location the decision to move an injured child (apart from the exceptions above) depends on how far you are from the nearest telephone, and how long it will take before medical assistance can get to you. Children weighing under 20kg (44lbs), whose injuries consist of fractures below the knee, may be carried for short distances provided the limb has been splinted and the patient experiences no discomfort.

ASSESSING THE SITUATION

Infants are particularly prone to choking and viral infections; toddlers and older children are prone to injuries received during play and as a result of their unstoppable fascination with the world around them. Whatever the situation in which you find yourself, the key to being an effective first responder is to follow the basic guidelines in the sequences recommended in this section.

Upon arrival at the scene of any accident, the competent first responder will endeavour to calmly sum up the situation by establishing the following vital facts in the shortest amount of time possible. Not only will this information guide your immediate course of action, it must also be relayed to any medical personnel that are called to the scene:

- What happened and how did it happen?
- How many persons (children) are injured?
- Is everyone, including the first responder and/or any other helpers, free from danger?
- Is medical assistance necessary?

THE 'SAFE' APPROACH

The **SAFE** acronym (below) summarizes the correct sequence in an easy-to-remember fashion. Whenever you approach a child that has collapsed, for any reason whatsoever, you should always:

- summon help immediately – either by yourself or by sending another reliable and responsible person to call for medical assistance while you begin to attend to the child.
- ensure your own safety as well as that of the child. This applies especially when attending to someone who has been injured in a traffic accident, fire or as a result of inhaling a toxic substance, as well as due to electric shock, or any other situation where the risk of injury persists in the vicinity.

WHEN A CHILD HAS COLLAPSED

Various injuries as well as medical conditions can cause a child to become confused and dazed in the more extreme cases he may even lose consciousness. If you are the first responder at a scene where a child has collapsed for unknown reasons, it is your duty to test the casualty's responsiveness (*see* opposite and page 14) to establish whether he is fully, or partly conscious

S **Shout for help:** Summon medical assistance or the emergency services immediately.

A **Approach with care:** Check for surrounding hazards that may also be a danger to yourself.

F **Free from danger:** Even though we recommend that casualties should not be moved, this precaution must be weighed against any obvious risk, e.g. if a child has been knocked down on a busy street you must move him or her – with all possible care, of course – to a safe place before commencing resuscitation.

E **Evaluate the ABC** (see page 18–21): Having taken the above precautions, you are now ready to assess vital functions and commence resuscitation if required.

or not. A temporary loss of consciousness occurs when the blood flow to the brain is decreased as a result of a sudden slowing of the heart rate. The condition commonly occurs when someone is feeling very hot, not eating enough, or as the result of emotional upset. Usually, the only first aid required is reassurance and something sweet to drink once consciousness returns.

The unconscious child

Check the responsiveness of a child lying motionless on the ground (*see* page 14 'ARE YOU ALRIGHT?') to establish that his airway is clear and that breathing and circulation are satisfactory. If the vital signs check out alright, then stay with the child to keep him calm until medical assistance arrives. If the child is very drowsy, position him in the recovery position (*see* page 23).

WHAT TO DO

- Check the response (as described above and on page 14). If there is no response, **call for help**.

- Your priority is to **check the ABC** (*see* page 18). If the airway is blocked the child will be unable to breathe so your aim is to **open the airway** (for children: *see* page 24; for infants: *see* page 27), check the breathing again and, if necessary, administer rescue breaths (for children: *see* page 24; for infants: *see* page 27).

- If the child is breathing and displays signs of life, such as coughing and movement, position him in the **recovery position** (for children: *see* page 23; for infants: *see* page 26).

- If the child has stopped breathing and shows no signs of life, immediately begin with **chest compressions** (for children: *see* page 25; for infants: *see* page 27).

Unconsciousness as a result of a near-drowning incident

Near-drowning victims (*see also* pages 96–99) may be unconscious and will probably be unable to breathe as a result of having been under water.

WHAT TO DO

- Get the child out of the water immediately.

- Call an ambulance. It is imperative that you get help in all cases of near-drowning.

- If the child is not breathing **commence rescue breathing** without delay (for children: *see* page 24; for infants: *see* page 27).

- When the child is breathing normally again, position him in the **recovery position** (for children: *see* page 23; for infants: *see* page 26).

UNCONSCIOUS WITH A SUSPECTED NECK INJURY

If there is ANY possibility of a neck injury in an unconscious child who is not breathing, you must restore breathing without moving the head. To do this you must apply the jaw-thrust method: if the child is breathing, kneel behind him and gently cup its head between your palms, thumbs resting on the cheek bones and fingers touching the jaw, keeping head, neck and body aligned. Stay with the child, reassure and calm him if he is frightened, and ask the child not to move. Continue to gently support the head in alignment with neck and body, until medical assistance arrives.

PROCEDURES FOR RESUSCITATION

To be really useful and effective, first aid procedures must adhere to certain rules and be performed in a specific sequence. This section outlines the basic skills and proven step-by-step techniques that you must follow. To become adept at these you should join a recognized first-aid course in your area, so that you can gain practical experience and become comfortable in the knowledge that you know what to do.

Normal breathing and blood circulation supply the body with oxygen and nutrients. These vital functions may become impaired, or fail completely during injury or acute illness, creating a serious condition that calls for immediate action.

Cardiopulmonary resuscitation (CPR) is a combination of rescue breathing and chest compressions designed to re-establish respiration and heartbeat. It consists of a practical set of skills that enable you to:
- ensure a clear airway
- assess adequacy of breathing and circulation
- provide oxygen to a child who is not breathing
- re-establish a heartbeat.

ESTABLISHING THE ABC
The ABC is what we focus on during all life-support procedures, and always in this sequence. It is very easy to remember this, the common purpose in life-support manoeuvres, as it ensures:

- **A**irway – the child has a clear anatomical channel through which to breathe.
- **B**reathing – oxygen can flow through the airway and into the lungs.
- **C**irculation – the blood carries oxygen from the lungs to all parts of the body.

Checking the airway
The airway extends from the mouth and nose down to the windpipe. A child's airway is narrower than an adult's – the smaller the child, the greater the risk of choking or suffocation. A child's airway may become obstructed by mucus; enlarged tonsils; food or solid matter that cannot be swallowed; and abnormal positioning of the head (as can happen if the child is unconscious).

The nerve reflex that stops food 'going down the wrong way' in adults is not completely developed in infants and toddlers, which is why they are so prone to **choking** (*see* page 28) and aspiration (that is, foreign objects going into the lungs).

A child's airway is also softer and more pliable than an adult's – therefore avoid compressing any part of

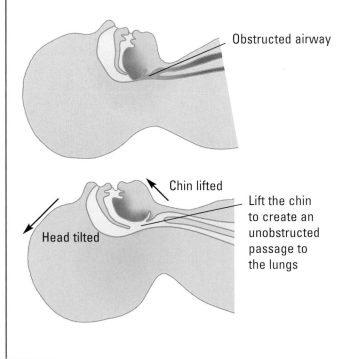

Obstructed airway

Chin lifted

Head tilted

Lift the chin to create an unobstructed passage to the lungs

the airway with your hands during resuscitation. Keep the child's head in a neutral position so that no part of the airway becomes stretched or kinked.

WHAT TO DO

- Check that there is no kinking of the windpipe due to abnormal positioning of the head.

- Check that the tongue has not fallen back into the throat (*see* **chin lift** page 18).

- That there is no obstruction by a foreign matter (*see* **choking** page 28).

Restoring breathing

Children breathe faster than adults – their bodies burn up oxygen at a faster rate. A child struggling to breathe will run out of energy sooner than an adult and may stop breathing quite suddenly when exhausted.

NORMAL BREATHING RATE IN CHILDREN	
Age (in years)	Breaths per minute
under 2 months	50 – 60
2 – 12 months	40 – 50
2 – 5 years	20 – 30
5 – 12 years	15 – 20
over 12 years	12 – 16

WHAT TO DO

- Restore the normal position of the tongue and the airway by using a combination of the **chin-lift and head-tilt** (for children: *see* page 24; for infants: *see* page 27).

- Carefully and gently feel in the mouth for foreign bodies and remove what you see (for children: *see* page 28; for infants: *see* page 30).

- When you have opened the airway the child may start breathing again spontaneously. If not, begin **rescue breathing** (for children: *see* page 24; for infants: *see* page 27).

- If the child begins to breathe unaided, place it in the recovery position (for children: *see* page 23; for infants: *see* page 26). Monitor its vital signs.

BREATHING DIFFICULTIES

The following are possible indicators that a child with breathing difficulty is in need of urgent medical attention:

- increasing rate of breathing (*see* table at left);
- noisy breathing or wheezing;
- visible flaring of the nostrils each time the child breathes in (in an infant, the use of these muscles may cause the head to bob up and down with each laboured intake of breath);
- sucking in of the muscles between the ribs each time the child breathes in;
- visible contraction of the neck muscles each time the child breathes in;
- the child's skin loses its healthy colour, turning mottled, dusky or pale;
- the skin, and fingers in particular, feel cold to your touch;
- the child has no interest in food or is too tired to eat or drink;
- the child becomes drowsy;
- rapid breathing suddenly slows, or becomes shallow.

Assessing the circulation

The smaller the child, the faster the normal heart rate. You can assess the state of the circulation most easily by feeling the pulse of the heartbeat transmitted through an artery that runs just under the skin (*see* **WHAT TO DO** on this page). The main reason for feeling the pulse is to measure the heart rate – that is, the number of beats per minute. Normally, the rate should fall within the ranges shown in the table below.

NORMAL HEART RATE IN CHILDREN	
Age (in years)	**Heartbeats per minute**
under 1 year	110 – 160
2 – 5 years	95 – 140
5 – 12 years	80 – 120
over 12 years	60 – 100

Faster-than-normal pulse rate
There are many reasons for a raised pulse rate in children, such as fever, excitement or distress. If the child is injured, however, a fast pulse rate should alert you to the possibility of **blood loss** or **shock** (*see* page 21).

Slower-than-normal pulse rate
A pulse rate below the normal ranges shown in the table above may indicate that the child is dangerously short of oxygen, and that the heart may soon stop beating altogether. Call a doctor or an ambulance immediately, and get ready to start basic life support.

Irregular pulse rate
A persistently irregular heartbeat indicates a medical problem that needs urgent attention. If a child is losing blood or is in shock for any other reason, the pulse in an artery becomes weak and may be difficult or even impossible to feel.

WHAT TO DO

- In infants and small children the pulse is easily felt in the **brachial artery** (crook of the arm), in older children in the **carotid artery** (side of the neck). In a healthy child, you can feel the pulse of the **radial artery** (inside of wrist). In a sick child, the pulse here is often too weak to be reliable.

- The rhythm of the pulse should be regular and strong enough for you to feel easily.

- If you cannot detect a pulse at all and the heart has stopped beating restore circulation without delay using rhythmic **chest compressions** (for children: *see* page 25; for infants: *see* page 27).

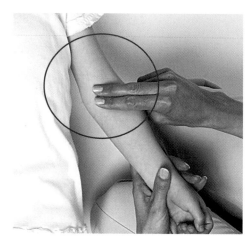

Location of the brachial artery inside the elbow.

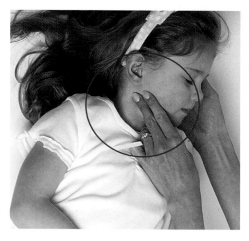

Location of carotid artery at the side of the neck.

PHYSICAL SIGNS THAT MAY INDICATE POOR CIRCULATION OR SHOCK

- The heart rate is faster or slower than the ranges indicated in the table on page 20.
- The pulse rhythm is irregular.
- The arterial pulse is weak or difficult to feel.
- The lips, tongue and mouth lining are pale or dusky instead of a healthy pink colour.
- The child's fingers are cold to your touch.
- The child becomes increasingly drowsy even in the absence of head injury.
- There is active bleeding from an injury to any part of the body.

What is 'shock'?

In medical terminology, 'shock' refers to any disorder of the blood circulation which interferes with the normal supply of oxygen and nutrients to the rest of the body, and in particular to the vital organs – the brain, kidneys, heart and lungs.

Bleeding and shock

Shock due to loss of blood requires urgent medical attention. In children, it most frequently results from injury to larger bones – particularly the pelvis – or to the liver and spleen, in which case bleeding may not be obvious at first glance. It is therefore vital that you assess the circulation to establish whether shock is developing, or already present.

Although a child's body can compensate for the effects of blood loss, in younger children these mechanisms can become exhausted quickly. When that happens blood pressure drops, putting the vital organs at risk. In addition to recognizing the early signs of shock in a bleeding child, it is also necessary to control blood loss while you wait for medical assistance.

Replacing fluid in shock: 'Mom, I'm thirsty!'

As a general rule, every injured child will complain of a dry mouth. This is part of the body's natural response to any form of injury – minor or major.

- If the child has a minor injury, offer him something to drink as a comfort rather than a necessity.

- If the child has been seriously injured, do not give him anything at all to eat or drink before he is assessed by a doctor.

WHAT TO DO

- Always call for help.

- Assess the child's ABC (pulse rate and volume, skin colour and temperature).

- Exert firm pressure over bleeding wounds, using a sterile or clean dressing fixed in place with sticking plaster. Covering open wounds helps to reduce the risk of infection.

- Splint fractured bones (*see* pages 49–51). Splinting reduces pain and the risk of sharp bone fragments damaging blood vessels and nerves.

- To divert blood to the vital organs, raise the child's legs higher than the rest of the body using a firm cushion or a rolled-up blanket.

- Keep the child covered to reduce heat loss.

RESUSCITATION FOR CHILDREN 1–8 YEARS

For each of the three 'What to do' scenarios on the following pages it is assumed that you have classified into the relevant and correct scenario. They may be categorized as follows:

1. Unconscious - breathing - sign of life

2. Unconscious - not breathing - sign of life

3. Unconscious - not breathing - no sign of life

The resuscitation procedure can be broken down into three major scenarios that you may encounter. It is important that you first assess which category the child falls into before you begin treating it.

Condition	Children 1–8 years of age
Unconscious breathing (*see* below)	Place in **recovery position** (*see* opposite) Call an ambulance Ensure airway remains open and that normal breathing continues
Unconscious not breathing signs of life/ circulation (*see* page 24)	Call an ambulance **Open the airway** (chin lift and head tilt – *see* page 24) Listen and look for signs of breathing for 10 seconds Give **2 effective rescue breaths** Check the **circulation** (*see* page 20) – refer to Scenario 3 (*see* page 25) if necessary
Unconscious not breathing no signs of life/ no circulation (*see* page 25)	No circulation: **5 chest compressions with 1 hand** Continue cycles of **1 breath to 5 chest compressions** Continue until normal breathing resumes of help arrives Place in recovery position if breathing resumes, and monitor carefully

SCENARIO 1   unconscious   breathing   signs of life/circulation

WHAT TO DO

- Place the child in the **recovery position** (*see* opposite).

- Call an ambulance.

- Ensure the airway remains open and that normal breathing continues.

UNCONSCIOUS CHILD (RECOVERY POSITION)

An unconscious child who is breathing unaided and has normal circulation should be placed in the recovery position. You need to put the child on her side to prevent the tongue from falling back, minimize the risk of vomit being sucked into the lungs and allow you to monitor her breathing and circulation as you wait for help. For treatment in case of suspected neck or spinal injury see page 55.

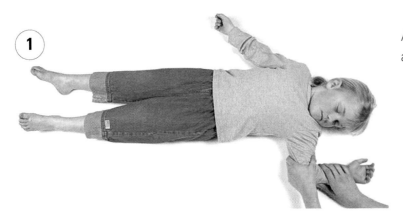

1 Angle the right arm next to the child's head at approximately 90°.

2 Position the right hand as shown and bring the left across her chest towards you to, palm showing out and the back of the hand resting against the right cheek. Bend the left leg at the knee as shown.

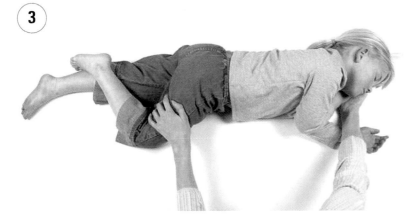

3 You can now move the child into the recovery position, your one hand stabilizing her head to protect her neck, while you use the other to bend her knee. Gently roll the trunk over. Ensure that her airway remains open and she continues to breathe normally.

SCENARIO 2   unconscious   not breathing   signs of life/circulation

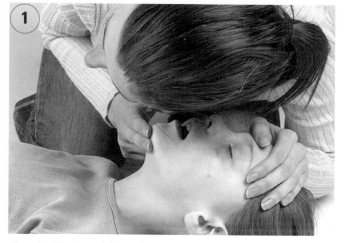

Gently lift the chin using two fingers of one hand while the other holds the head steady. Listen and feel for signs of breathing for 10 seconds.

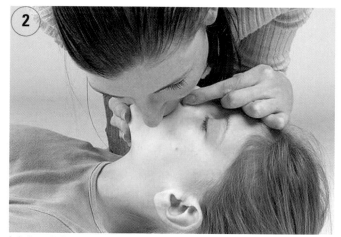

Maintaining the chin lift and position of the head, gently pinch the nose shut with the fingers of your other hand and inhale.

To use a **face shield**: place it over the child's face, filter in the mouth. Pinch its nose shut and breathe directly through the filter.

WHAT TO DO

- Call an ambulance.

- **Open the airway** using chin lift and head tilt (*see* step 1).

- Listen and look for **signs of breathing** for about 10 seconds.

- If there is no sign of breathing, open casualty's mouth, pinch his nose shut and **administer 2 effective rescue breaths** (*see* step 3).

- **Check the circulation**.

- Continue rescue breaths at a rate of 1 every 3 seconds (20 per minute) until the child begins to breathe unaided or help arrrives. Check the circulation every minute.

- Place the child in the **recovery position** if she begins to breathe normally.

- If you are alone, give 2 effective rescue breaths then call an ambulance.

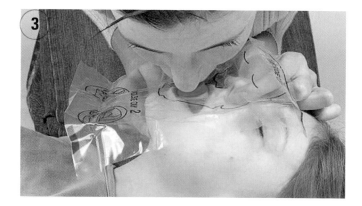

SCENARIO 3   unconscious   not breathing   no signs of life/circulation

WHAT TO DO

- Call an ambulance.

- Open the airway (*see* opposite, step 1) and make 5 attempts to give **2 effective rescue breaths** (*see* opposite, step 3).

- Position your hand over the lower half of the breast-bone as shown (right) and do **5 compressions using only the heel of one hand**. Keeping your arm straight, lean over the child and press down on the child's chest. Keep your fingers lifted. Do compressions at a rate of 100 per minute.

- You must give **1 effective rescue breath between every 5 compressions** and continue until breathing resumes or medical help arrives.

- Place in **recovery position** if casualty begins to breathe unaided.

- If you are alone: cycles of 1 breath to 5 compressions for one minute, then call an ambulance.

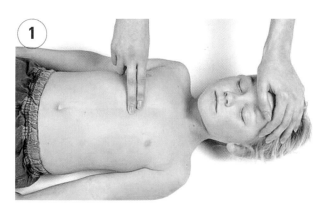

Locate the child's lowest rib. Trace the line of this rib to where it meets the breastbone. Position your middle finger on this spot, resting your index finger on the lowest rib.

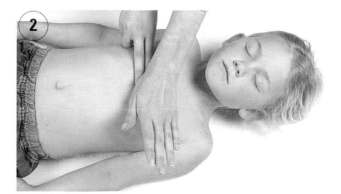

Position the heel of your other hand next to your two fingers, over the lower part of the breastbone. You only use the heel of your hand to do chest compressions on a child.

Using the heel of one hand only, compress the chest to a depth of about 3cm (1in) in a quick movement. For every 5 chest compressions, give 1 effective rescue breath. Do 100 compressions per minute, alternating with rescue breaths as described. Do this until the child is breathing spontaneously, or until medical help arrives.

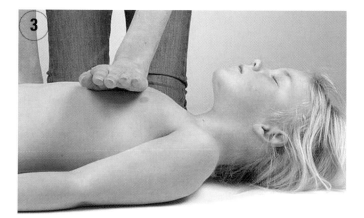

RESUSCITATION FOR INFANTS UP TO 12 MONTHS

The resuscitation procedure can be broken down into three major scenarios that you may encounter. It is important that you first assess which category the infant falls into before you begin treating it.

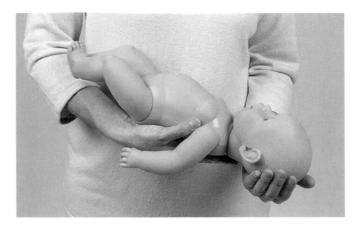

RECOVERY POSITION

Cradle the infant in your arms. Your one hand should support his head, holding it slightly below the rest of the body, while the other hand firmly supports the infant's back.

Condition	Infants 0–12 months of age
Unconscious breathing (*see* below)	Hold in **recovery position** (*see* below) Call an ambulance Ensure airway remains open and normal breathing continues
Unconscious not breathing signs of life/ circulation (*see* opposite)	Call an ambulance **Open the airway** (chin lift and head tilt – *see* opposite) Listen and look for signs of breathing for 10 seconds Give **2 effective rescue breaths** Check the **circulation** (*see* page 20) – refer to Scenario 3 (*see* opposite) if necessary
Unconscious not breathing no signs of life/ no circulation (*see* opposite)	If no circulation give **5 chest compressions using 2 fingers** Continue cycles of **1 breath to 5 chest compressions** Continue until normal breathing resumes or help arrives If normal breathing resumes place in recovery position (*see* above) and monitor carefully

SCENARIO 1 unconscious breathing signs of life/circulation

WHAT TO DO

- Place the infant in the **recovery position** (*see* top).

- Call an ambulance.

- Ensure the airway remains open and that normal breathing continues.

SCENARIO 2   unconscious   not breathing   signs of life/circulation

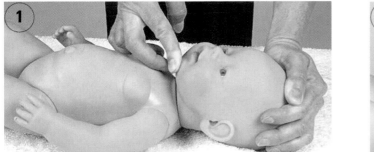
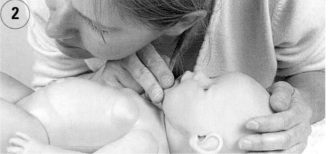

With one hand stabilize the infant's head. Tilt his chin up with the index finger of your other hand to open the airway. Listen for sounds of breathing for 10 seconds. Then cover mouth and nose with yours and gently exhale.

WHAT TO DO
- Call an ambulance.

- Open the airway; give **2 effective rescue breaths** (*see* right); check the circulation.

- Do rescue breaths at a rate of 1 breath every 3 seconds (20 per minute) until infant starts to breathe or help arrives. Check the circulation every minute.

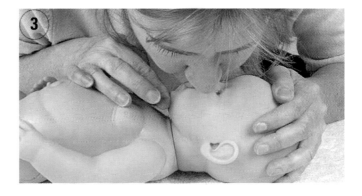

- If you are alone, give 2 effective rescue breaths then call an ambulance.

- When the infant begins to breathe unaided, hold in recovery position (*see* opposite page, top).

SCENARIO 3   unconscious   not breathing   no signs of life/circulation

WHAT TO DO
- Call an ambulance.

- Open airway and **give 2 effective rescue breaths**.

- **Using 2 fingers do 5 chest compressions** (at a rate of 100 per minute) to a depth of about 2cm (3/4in). Give **1 effective rescue breath for every 5 compressions** until breathing resumes or help arrives.

- Alone: do one minute of 1 breath per 5 compressions. Call ambulance, taking the infant with you.

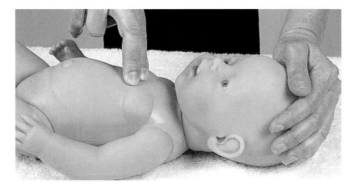

Position the infant on a firm flat surface. Trace a line between the infant's nipples and put your two fingertips on a spot about a finger below that line.

CHOKING

Choking results when the upper airway is obstructed, commonly as a result of food or a small object becoming impacted. In some cases, a coughing spell may be enough to expel the foreign body and clear the airway. However, even small objects can lodge firmly in the narrow airway of an infant or small child, in which case you may have to use the techniques described on these pages.

Object in the nostril

Object in back of throat

Tongue

Food stuck in throat

Oesophagus (to gullet)

Trachea (to windpipe)

FIRST AID FOR CHOKING CHILDREN 1–8 YEARS

Condition	Children 1–8 years of age
Suspected choking	Up to 5 back blows – check the mouth and remove any obstruction Up to 5 chest thrusts – check the mouth and remove any obstruction Up to 5 abdominal thrusts – check the mouth and remove any obstruction Do 3 cycles of back blows, chest thrusts and abdominal thrusts If breathing: **open airway** and remove visible foreign matter (*see* page 24) place in **recovery position** (*see* page 23) If not breathing, commence **resuscitation sequence** (*see* page 25)

Use a combination of back blows, chest thrusts and abdominal thrusts for small children who show signs of choking and are unable to breathe or cough up the foreign body themselves. **Do 3 cycles of the entire procedure then call an ambulance if there is no improvement**. Follow this with 5 attempts to give 2 effective rescue breaths. If still unsuccessful, begin resuscitation (*see* pages 22–25). You can stand, sit or kneel behind the child to perform these procedures.

BACK BLOWS – WHAT TO DO

- Stand or knee behind the child.

- Give up to five sharp back blows between the shoulder blades with the heel of your hand.

- Check the mouth for any obstructions and remove without probing blindly.

- If there is no relief, do 5 chest thrusts.

CHEST THRUSTS – WHAT TO DO

- If the back blows fail to clear the obstruction, do up to 5 chest thrusts.

- Make a fist and cover it with your other hand. Place against the lower part of the breastbone. Now press inwards sharply up to five times.

- Carefully check the mouth and remove any visible obstructions.

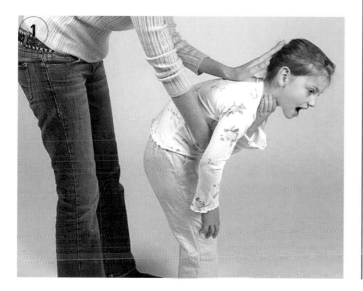

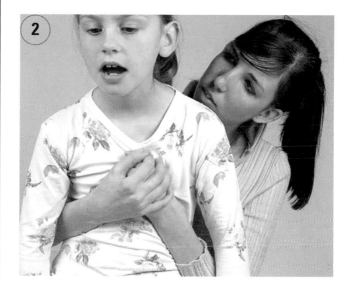

ABDOMINAL THRUSTS – WHAT TO DO

- If chest thrusts are ineffective in clearing the obstruction, do up to 5 abdominal thrusts.

- Place one fist on the child's abdomen, cover it with your free palm and then thrust firmly inwards and upwards up to five times.

- If the casualty begins to breathe again unaided, carefully check the mouth and clear away any visible foreign object.

- If there is no relief after 3 cycles of back blows, chest and abdominal thrusts **call an ambulance**.

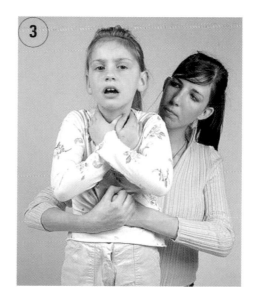

FIRST AID FOR CHOKING INFANTS 1–12 MONTHS

Condition	Infants 0–12 months of age
Suspected choking	Up to 5 back blows – check the mouth and remove any obstruction Up to 5 chest thrusts – check the mouth and remove any obstruction Do 3 cycles of back blows and chest thrusts If breathing: **open airway** and remove visible foreign matter (*see* page 26) hold in **recovery position** (*see* page 26) If not breathing, commence **resuscitation sequence** (*see* page 27)

Use a combination of back blows and chest thrusts for choking infants. **Do 3 cycles of the entire procedure, then call an ambulance if there is no improvement**. Follow with 5 attempts to give 2 effective rescue breaths. If unsuccessful, begin resuscitation (*see* pages 26–7). **NOTE: NEVER DO ABDOMINAL THRUSTS ON AN INFANT.**

BACK BLOWS – WHAT TO DO

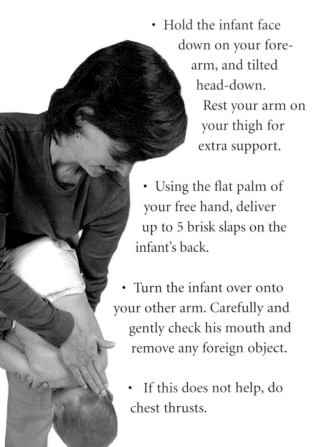

• Hold the infant face down on your forearm, and tilted head-down. Rest your arm on your thigh for extra support.

• Using the flat palm of your free hand, deliver up to 5 brisk slaps on the infant's back.

• Turn the infant over onto your other arm. Carefully and gently check his mouth and remove any foreign object.

• If this does not help, do chest thrusts.

CHEST THRUSTS – WHAT TO DO

• Turn the infant face-up, with his head lower than his hips, supported on your forearm.

• With the tips of two fingers, give 5 chest thrusts over the breastbone (depress about 2cm; ¾in). Thrusts should be aimed downwards and be about three seconds apart.

• Check the mouth. If the infant does not breathe after 3 cycles, call an ambulance immediately.

NEVER DO ABDOMINAL THRUSTS ON AN INFANT

SAFETY IN THE HOME

Your home should be a place of happiness, your sanctuary, a shelter from the elements and a place where your personal history will unfold as your family grows. Accidents can – and do – happen, but you can lower the odds considerably by applying a few general safety precautions. No hi-tech equipment is needed; all you need to safeguard the happiness and health of your family is dedication, vigilance and some common sense.

The majority of childhood accidents occur in and around the home – the place we think is safest. This is hardly surprising. Home is where children spend most of their early lives, begin to move about and discover the world around them – finding out how it looks, feels, tastes, smells and sounds. This incredible journey of discovery is one that even the most docile child must undertake. The little rascal who scurries around the living room grabbing, tugging and sticking everything into his mouth is often labelled 'naughty', but this behaviour is a vital part of his normal development.

We cannot stop our children from finding things out for themselves – and of course we should not. This section will help you see your home with new eyes and recognize common hazards for the developing child. It discusses some basic safety devices and strategies for minimizing the risk of injury while still allowing your growing child the much-needed freedom to explore.

A NOTE

The measures listed in this book are by no means the last word on child safety, and no single safety tip should be regarded as a guarantee against injury. You can obtain more detailed information about commercially available safety devices and child safety training courses for parents and child minders from the child safety or general accident prevention organizations operating in your country. Some with proven track records are listed on page 158.

Your adventurous child needs supervision to keep him out of trouble. For all children, particularly infants and toddlers, the most important safety device is the one you cannot buy – the watchful eye of a responsible adult. Think of it as SUPER VISION – your eye always on the child, whatever tasks you may be juggling, even if the doorbell chimes, the phone rings and the pot on the stove boils over all at the same time. Never leave your infant or child alone anywhere.

If you are still planning your family, the quickest way to identify safety hazards in your home is to invite a friend or family member to bring her own one-year-old bundle of joy over and let her loose. Within an hour you will know exactly where the problems areas are. But if your nerves are not made of tempered steel, following these 10 suggestions might be less harrowing.

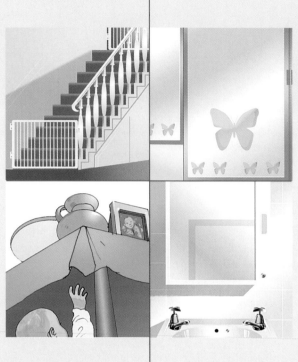

1 Do not throw anything that might be harmful to your child into an open bin or container. Assume that your child, particularly when he is at the crawling stage, will be fascinated by whatever the bin holds and want to shove it directly into his mouth.

2 Store poisonous substances in locked cupboards or on high shelves that cannot be reached – in the lounge (liquor cabinets), kitchen, bathroom and garage or workshop.

3 Make sure that all poisonous or harmful substances are packaged in bottles or containers which are clearly labelled with stickers. Never decant poisons into old food or drink containers while there are small children in the home. Ask your pharmacist to dispense all medicines and tablets in childproof containers, and keep these in a wall-mounted medicine chest out of children's reach.

4 Avoid table covers that a toddler may tug, bringing everything on the tabletop crashing down.

5 Keep sharp items such as scissors, letter openers and metal kitchen utensils out of sight and out of reach, preferably in locked drawers.

6 Prevent infants and toddlers from gaining access to solid foodstuffs, toy parts or any objects small enough to fit into their mouths, noses or ears. The smaller the child, the less able she is to spit or cough them out, so there is a high risk of airway obstruction, choking and suffocation. For this reason too the toddler's toys should be the right kind for her age, with no small parts that come off, and not made of materials that might be poisonous if chewed. Only buy toys tested and approved by the national standards bureau operating in your country.

7 Keep matches, lighters and burning cigarettes well away from children. (And keep unlit cigarettes away from them too.)

8 Block off all staircases by installing safety gates at the top and bottom. These should comply with national standards for their height and the spacing of their bars – not more than 6cm (2½ in) apart. These gates can be removed once your youngest child is walking confidently enough to negotiate stairs without danger.

9 Mark large panes of glass in windows or doors with bright stickers. Small children at play may become so absorbed in chasing each other around the house that they will not notice the difference between glass and fresh air.

10 Never carry a cup of tea or any other hot liquid in one hand while using the other hand to hold, carry or nurse a baby or small child. The time you save by 'multi-tasking' is not worth the risk of stumbling and scalding the child.

SETTING A GOOD EXAMPLE

Like all other habits (good and bad), children learn safe behaviour from their significant role models – older siblings, teachers and, most of all, you, the parent. If you wear a seat belt without fail you will have no trouble getting your children to do the same. To punish children for taking the same risks they have seen you take regularly is not only counterproductive, it confuses them, and eats away at the trust which is such an important element of family relationships. So try to set a good example.

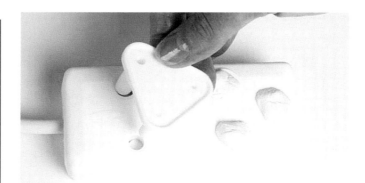

Whether you use two- or three-pronged plugs, cover unused points to deter prying fingers.

Electrical safety

Particularly if your house is more than 25 years old, ask an electrical contractor to check the wiring and to ensure that the circuit-breakers are functioning properly. In addition, ask your electrician to install as many power points as you need in any room or space, rather than mounting multi-plug adaptors on top of one another. Keep exposed wiring and extension cords to a minimum, and ensure that the insulation layer is not frayed or cracked at any point.

Do not buy any electrical appliances that have not been approved by the testing authority in your country. These are seldom properly tested, or adapted for the electrical supply in your country. As a result, they may overheat, or damage the electrical circuits in your home. What appears at first to be a bargain may cost a lot more in the long run, as well as being hazardous to your family.

Make sure that supply cords from table lamps, kettles and other appliances are only as long as is

necessary, and that they are well concealed. Small children just love to give these a yank. Why? To see what will happen, of course!

Cover all unused electric power points. Inexpensive safety covers are available from child safety organizations and electrical retailers. Alternatively, unconnected two-point or three-point plugs secured in place with a blob of mouldable non-toxic adhesive will do just as well.

Unplug any household electric appliance that is not in use and store it in a safe place. Switch off all electric power points not in use.

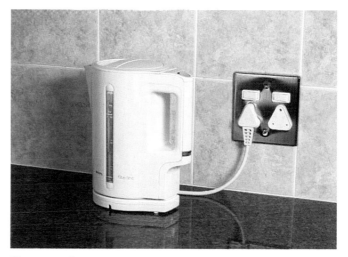

Keep appliance cords short and out of reach.

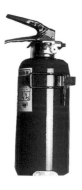

Fire safety

Fire in the home is one of a parent's greatest fears, and so it should be. It threatens life and limb of the entire family and has the power to destroy everything you hold dear, in an instant. It can start at any point in the home where enough heat is generated – from unprotected flames, defective or overloaded electrical circuits, the stove, leaking gas that ignites, or heaters standing too close to flammable materials. Besides this, non-flammable materials that do not actually ignite when heated can still generate enough smoke to cause serious injury or death from inhalation of smoke or toxic chemicals.

Safety tips: dealing with fire hazards at home

- Install a wall-mounted fire extinguisher in your kitchen, at a level where children cannot reach it, and get it serviced regularly.
- Install fireguards (below) around open wood, coal or gas fires. Do not hang clothing or anything else on the fireguard – this only creates another fire hazard.
- Fit at least one approved smoke detector per level in a multi-storey house. In a single-level house, install the detector just outside your kitchen. Check the batteries at least once a year.

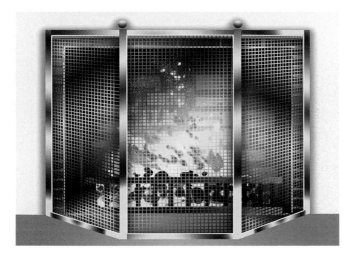

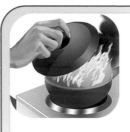

POTS ON FIRE

If hot oil on your stove bursts into flame, do not move the pot or pour water over it, and do not attack it with the fire extinguisher – this will just cause burning oil to splash everywhere. Cover the pot with a snug-fitting lid or wooden breadboard to kill the flames by starving them of oxygen, and switch off the gas or power supply. Do not disturb the pot until it has completely cooled. Consider baking potato chips in the oven instead – it is healthier and safer!

- Avoid electric bar heaters and space heaters, which are difficult to child-proof. Closed-system heaters fuelled by gas, anthracite or oil are safer.
- Clean ovens regularly so there is no old dripped food in them that might catch fire.
- Ban smoking in bedrooms (and preferably everywhere indoors).
- Train children to keep their distance from heaters and open fires, particularly if their night clothes are made of flammable materials.
- Do not light outdoor fires closer than 5m (15ft) to your house. Avoid open outdoor fires when the wind is blowing, particularly in dry weather. Never coax a smouldering fire by pouring lighter fuel or any other flammable liquid over it.
- Designate one outside door as the best escape route in the event of fire. If the worst happens, grab your children, cover their mouths and noses with handkerchiefs or other material to reduce smoke inhalation, and get out.

Water safety

Children love playing with water – it attracts them like a magical force. Next time you enjoy a summer's day at the beach, look out for any young mother with a toddler. You will see how she battles to keep her little bundle of energy from charging off toward the water's edge again and again – and you will understand that where water is concerned, the cardinal safety rule is SUPERVISION. Nothing substitutes for an adult's watchful eye.

Never leave small children alone near water – a fish pond, splash pool, lake or the sea – or even a full washing bucket. It does not matter if the water is shallow at all points. Small children can drown in water no deeper than 2.5cm (1in) – just enough to cover the mouth and nose.

Even children who have been taught to swim should be closely supervised in water until the age of eight. Smaller children should never enter a swimming pool enclosure without a flotation device, even if you are holding them in the pool. Whatever device you prefer to use should be snug-fitting, age-appropriate, and approved by your national standards authority. Children under 12 months of age lose heat very quickly in unheated water and should not be in a pool for more than 15 minutes at a time.

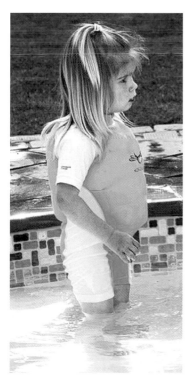
Flotation devices are essential for small children.

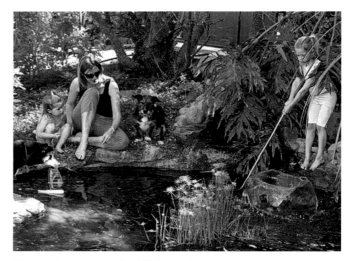
Never leave small children alone near water.

Swimming pool safety

In most countries it is a legal requirement to provide secure fencing around domestic swimming pools, and to ensure that the enclosure satisfies set measurements and other criteria. The following specifications are common to legislation in almost all countries where such laws are in place, but please check with your local authority or county council that your fence is 100% in keeping with the regional or national laws or by-laws.

- All swimming pool fences should be 1.2m (4ft) in height at all points, with no gaps of more than 10cm (4in) above ground level.
- Gaps between vertical poles should be no more than 10cm (4in).
- Gates should be the same height as the fence, automatically self-closing and self-latching, and open outward (away from the pool) to prevent children pushing their way through an unlatched gate.
- Gate latches should be a minimum of 1.2m (4ft) from the ground if on the inside of the gate and 1.5m (5ft) from the ground if on the outside.
- Gates should always be closed.
- There should be nothing near or leaning against the pool fence to tempt children to climb over.

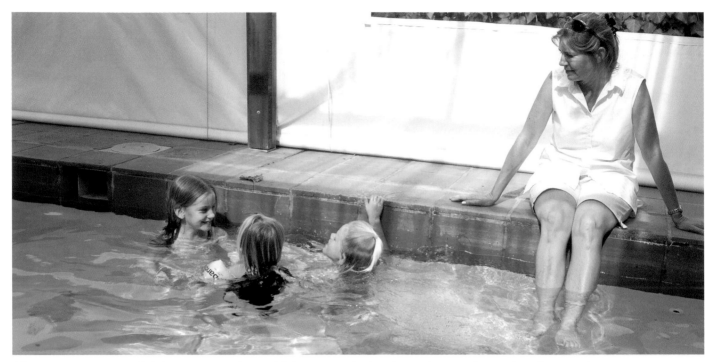

Always ensure an adult is present when children are playing in and around a swimming pool.

- Pool nets and covers are not a substitute for adult supervision or proper fences. Non-permeable pool covers collect rainwater and may themselves become drowning hazards.
- Do not permit children to play games inside a fenced swimming pool enclosure.
- Inflatable pools should be emptied immediately after use and deflated. All other portable pools should be stored upside down when not in use.

Buy only pool chemicals with childproof lids. Store them in a secure cupboard or tool shed, and not next to the pool. All pool chemicals are highly concentrated and lethal if swallowed.

If you install a swimming pool or a spa in your home, be prepared to deal with water accidents. Read the chapters on basic life support (*see* pages 16–30), and take a recognized CPR (cardiopulmonary resuscitation) course. Remember, quick action saves lives. If your child goes missing from the house, check the pool first.

Bathroom safety

The bathroom can be a very risky place, especially for small children whose inquisitive natures can lead to all sorts of unforeseen mishaps and disasters. Follow these sensible tips to protect your child against scalding, falls on hard, slippery surfaces, and drowning.

- Fill bath tubs only as deep as necessary in order to wash the child.
- When you are filling the bath tub, run the cold water before the hot, not hot first or both at the same time.
- Always check the bathwater temperature carefully before placing the child in the tub.
- Set the hot water thermostats of your hot water geyser to a maximum of 54°C (120°F) to prevent the risk of scalding.
- Position your child so that you can wash him at the end furthest away from taps – to prevent hot water dripping onto the child.

- Place a non-slip rubber mat in the tub.
- Discourage toddlers from standing in the tub.
- There should be no portable electrical appliances or unprotected electrical sockets in the bathroom.
- And once again, do not leave small children alone in the bath tub, not even for a second.

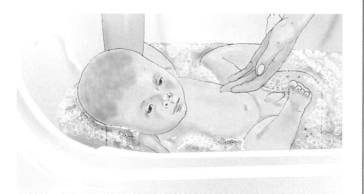

To prevent accidents, always place a non-slip rubber mat in a bath for babies or small children.

Kitchen safety

For many families, the kitchen is the heart of the home, particularly in the colder months. You may often have to prepare food or wash dishes while keeping an eye on children. If you follow these recommendations your child will be able to share the aromas and excitement of kitchen activity without being exposed to risk.

- High chairs keep infants and toddlers out of danger while allowing them to remain close to you in the kitchen. Ensure the child is securely harnessed in the chair to prevent him slipping under the tray and falling out.
- When cooking food, keep pot and pan handles turned away from the edge of the stove (right), and if possible use the back rings or plates.
- Store knives and other sharp cutlery and glass and breakable crockery in cupboards that are well out of

a small child's reach. Any floor-level cupboards which contain dangerous or poisonous items should be self-locking or fitted with secure child-proof latches.

- Keep plastic shopping bags, garbage bags and any other plastic sheeting collected for recycling locked away well out of children's reach to prevent accidental suffocation.
- Kettles should ideally be cordless or have the shortest possible cords, which are less likely to droop over the edge of the kitchen counter.

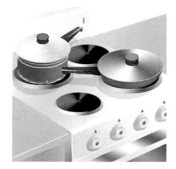

Be cautious about using microwave ovens, or allowing children to use them, to heat food or drinks. If unsure of how long to heat the food, or what power setting to use, always err on the side of caution. Lukewarm food may not be all that palatable, but a burnt mouth is agony! Always use appropriate containers that do not absorb too much heat. Before serving the food, stir it well to distribute heat evenly, and taste a mouthful yourself before serving it to your child.

SKIN AND SOFT-TISSUE INJURIES

Many minor injuries can be treated at home and require little more than a first-aid kit. Minor skin wounds that are correctly treated usually heal quickly, and with hardly any scarring. Cuts, scrapes and bruises are common as long as there are children of any age in the home, leading healthy, active lives. These injuries may be caused by sharp objects (kitchen equipment, tools, and so on), bites, falls, or bumps against solid objects.

BUMPS AND BRUISES

A bruise (or haematoma) can occur from a fall onto a hard surface, bumps against walls or furniture, or the blow of a cricket bat or ball. Although the skin is not broken, the blunt, high-energy impact ruptures small veins, causing mild bleeding – the greyish-brown blotch you see under the skin. As the dead blood cells are broken down by the body's natural defences, the bruise changes colour from brown to green and yellow over five to seven days, before disappearing completely within seven to 10 days.

➕ **FIRST AID**   Limit bleeding and swelling by immediately applying a cold compress (ice blocks wrapped in a cloth, or a bag of frozen peas) to the injured area. Give a mild painkiller such as paracetamol (acetaminophen) if the bruise begins to throb. Unless the overlying skin is broken, bruises rarely become infected, and dressings are of little benefit.

MAKING A COLD COMPRESS

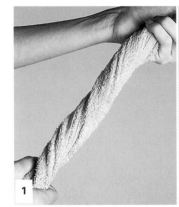
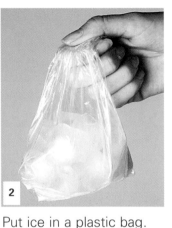

Wet and wring a towel.   Put ice in a plastic bag.

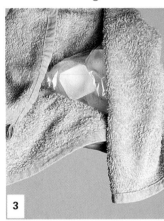
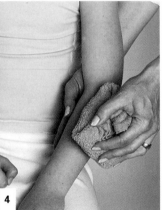

Wrap ice in the towel.   Apply to injured area.

Dark-skinned children may be more prone to the formation of keloid scars, which are prominent, and often out of proportion to the extent of the injury, even where treatment has been fault-less. It is usually not possible to prevent keloid formation, but steroid injections or cosmetic surgery may be helpful for scars which are very large or unsightly.

A black eye

This is most often caused by a sporting injury or a punch. The blunt impact causes rapid bruising around the eye, particularly in the eyelid, which often swells to obscure the eye completely.

FIRST AID The bruising may be reduced by immediately applying a cold compress to the eye socket for a few minutes. However, it is more important to ensure that the eye and the surrounding bone are not damaged. Any child with bruising covering up the eye should be examined by a doctor. (*See also* Eye Injuries, pages 57–59.)

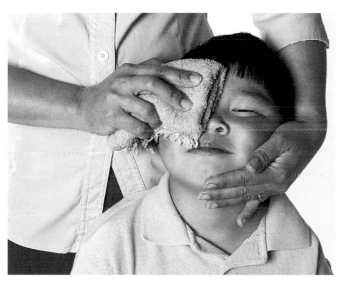

A cold compress reduces swelling and bruising.

Bruised fingernails

Bruising can occur under a fingernail or toenail (sub-ungual haematoma) crushed between hard surfaces or objects. Blood collects under the nail, which turns an unsightly blue-black colour. Because the blood supply to the base of the nail is often disturbed, the nail will usually fall off over time and be replaced by a new one.

Treating a bruised fingernail

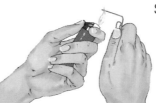

Straighten a paperclip, leaving one right-angle bend. Heat one end over a flame until it glows red-hot.

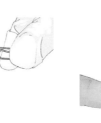

Press the hot end of the clip gently on the middle of the blackened nail. When you feel the nail 'give', remove the clip and allow blood to escape through the hole.

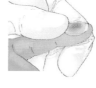

Massage the nail gently to improve drainage. Note: there is no value in performing this procedure more than once.

FIRST AID Bruised fingernails do not usually need medical attention. However, you can reduce the chance of the nail being lost by draining the blood out, using the easy, painless method shown above. The sooner you drain the blood, the more likely the nail is to survive.

Children who bruise easily

Few perfectly healthy children survive childhood without some bruises. However, be concerned about any child who seems to bruise very easily or often, or where the bruise is bigger than you would expect from the injury. A small number of children have inherited bleeding disorders or skin abnormalities that predispose to easy or excessive bruising, even after minor injuries. If your child fits this description, seek a medical opinion as soon as possible. (*See also* Blood Spots under the Skin, page 135.)

Always seek medical attention for:

- scalp bruises in babies and small children, as there is a possibility of underlying skull fracture;
- bruises with severe pain on movement, suggesting a possible underlying fracture;
- a black eye (bruising around the eye socket);
- straddle injuries, with bruising to the thighs and genital area (the bruise can become quite large, compressing the bladder outlet and making it difficult for the child to urinate);
- children who appear to bruise easily or excessively after a minor injury.

OPEN WOUNDS

Open wounds are ones where there is a break in the skin. Once the skin barrier is disturbed, bacteria can invade and there is a risk of infection. To prevent infection, you need to clean germs and dirt out of the wound, and keep them out, so your first-aid priority is to treat all open wounds as quickly and thoroughly as possible with simple hygienic measures: washing, cleaning and dressing.

FIRST AID **Step 1: Washing**

Bleeding is the body's own way of washing germs and dirt out of a fresh wound. The first-aid provider's task is to continue the good work by washing with water and a dilute antiseptic solution (for example, Savlon™, Dettol™ or similar). Even if you cannot see dirt particles in the wound, assume they are there and need to be washed out. Injured arms, legs, hands or feet can be washed easily and adequately under a cold-water tap. Simply let the running water wash freely over the wound for two minutes. Wounds on all parts of the body can be washed with cotton wool, or a clean cloth dipped in weak antiseptic solution.

Pure concentrated antiseptic is very painful when applied to raw wounds; it should always be diluted according to the manufacturer's instructions.

Bear in mind that the red pigment inside blood cells (haemoglobin) acts like a strong dye, so that even 5ml (a teaspoonful) of blood will colour a basin of water red. Unless blood is pumping quickly out of the wound, try not to let this dramatic picture worry you or your child too much. If the wound continues to bleed briskly after washing, apply direct pressure to it for two minutes with one or two clean gauze pads before proceeding to the next step.

Step 2: Cleaning

Each tiny particle of dirt or foreign matter increases the risk of infection in an open wound. Dirt left in it may also cause permanent 'tattooing' underneath the new layer of skin. So your second task is to carefully remove all dirt or foreign matter visible in the wound after washing.

First wipe the wound gently but firmly with a clean soft kitchen sponge dipped in dilute antiseptic solution. Then, using a clean pair of tweezers from your first-aid kit, pick out any ingrained dirt which remains. Scan the entire wound carefully – particularly if it is a large abrasion – for bits of soil, clothing or any foreign matter which can be easily removed without tugging or causing the child excessive pain.

Wounds with deeply ingrained soil or dirt which is difficult to remove in this way might require cleaning under a general anaesthetic. In such cases, cover the wound with a clean dressing and take the child to the nearest clinic or hospital.

Cleaning and dressing a wound

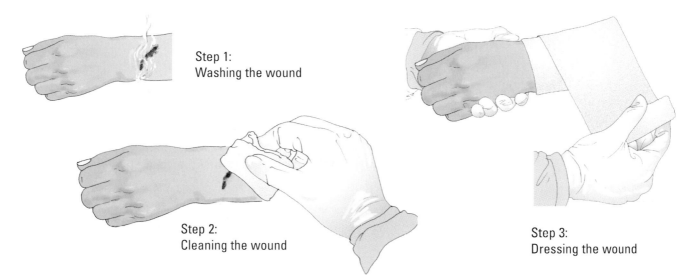

Step 1:
Washing the wound

Step 2:
Cleaning the wound

Step 3:
Dressing the wound

Step 3: Dressing

The main purpose of a dressing is to protect a fresh wound from re-injury, or becoming dirty or infected as the child resumes a normal level of activity. Tiny cuts and abrasions that are not actively bleeding may safely be left open, lightly dabbed with mercurochrome (no longer approved by the Food and Drug Administration in the United States) or antiseptic ointment or cream (for example, Savlon™, Dettol™ or Betadine™). But your child may insist you cover it with an adhesive plaster (for example, Band-Aid™) which will promptly be shown off to friends as proof of immense courage!

What to use

Most dressings have two components: a non-sticky pad or swab to cover the wound, and a secure bandage or adhesive plaster to keep the pad in place. Paraffin-impregnated gauze (Jelonet™) is a versatile dressing for any raw surface of skin. It conforms to the shape of the body surface, and comes away easily when removed. A single layer of paraffin gauze is sufficient to cover most wounds.

Do not use cotton wool to dress raw wounds because the fibres will become embedded in the scab, and removal may be very painful.

Do not encircle a finger, arm or leg with any tight plaster or bandage which could interfere with the blood supply. If the child complains of persistent pain, this could indicate that the dressing is too tight and it should be removed immediately.

Persistently brisk bleeding may be caused by a torn artery. If bleeding does not stop with direct pressure, cover the wound with a thick dressing secured with adhesive plaster, and take the child to your family doctor, or to hospital.

What size should the dressing be?

The dressing need only be big enough to cover the wound, and thick enough to remain dry (free of blood) on the surface. The bulkier the dressing, the more likely it is to come loose and need replacing within minutes or hours.

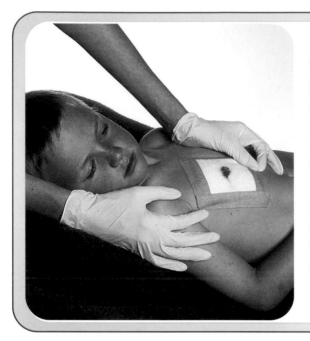

Whether you manage to clean a wound as described on page 40 will depend on how co-operative the child is. All soft-tissue injuries hurt, but each child experiences pain in his own individual way. Never feel obliged to try to cope on your own with a child who cannot be consoled, or struggles against you. It is better for all concerned to cover the wound with a clean dressing, and seek the assistance of a doctor or nurse. Let them deal with the injury, while you focus your energy on providing reassurance and comfort to the child.

Lotions

Spread a layer of antiseptic cream or ointment over abraded or raw skin before applying the dressing, which will prevent it sticking to the wound and make removal easier. If you have no medicated creams or ointments, a dab of plain petroleum jelly (Vaseline™) will do as well.

Never apply any powdered substances, foodstuffs or household cleaning agents to an open wound. Use only what is recommended here, or else nothing at all.

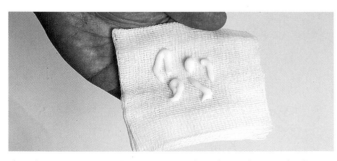

Apply antiseptic ointment to the dressing to help prevent infection.

Keeping the wound dry

Do your best to keep a fresh wound free of moisture for at least 48 hours.

How long do I leave the dressing on?

There is no hard-and-fast rule about how long a dressing should remain in place. You need not change it every day; doing so will disturb the scab, causing unnecessary discomfort and bleeding and delaying healing. However, a dressing that becomes wet, dirty, blood-soaked or tattered should be replaced. Dressings that remain clean and intact can be removed after seven days, and only replaced if the wound still appears raw.

How do I remove the dressing?

Many children dread this more than anything else. Your child may insist on removing the dressing herself. Let her do it if she wants to – even if it takes her a long time. If a dressing sticks fast to the wound, simply let her soak it in the bath tub for about 15 minutes. It will probably float off, or come away with a gentle tug.

SCRAPES AND ABRASIONS

An abrasion is a scrape that has shaved off some outer layers of the skin, and is deep enough to cause bleeding. Because tiny nerve endings just under the skin are damaged by the injury, abrasions can be particularly painful, depending on their size and depth.

✚ FIRST AID   Wash and clean abrasions as described on page 40 to reduce the chance of infection and 'tattooing'. If the scrape occurred through the child's clothing, or on a sandy or grimy surface, fabric or dirt will be embedded in the damaged skin.

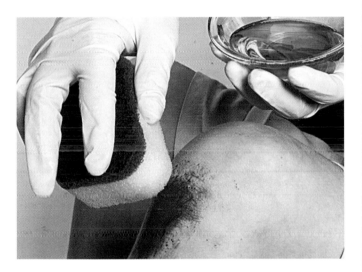

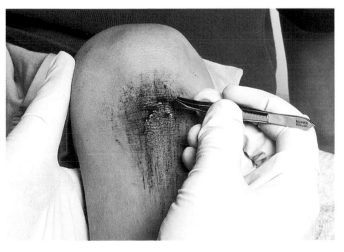

⊕ Always seek medical attention if:

- the child requires an anti-tetanus booster (*see* Tetanus, page 46);
- there is excessive bleeding;
- there is deeply ingrained dirt in the wound;
- the wound is too painful for you to clean adequately.

Lacerations

A child's skin is delicate and can easily be lacerated (cut or torn) by sharp objects or blunt impact.

✚ FIRST AID   Wash and clean the wound as indicated on page 40. If a flap of skin has been lifted over the cut, wash and clean well underneath the flap. If necessary, reduce or stop bleeding by applying pressure with a clean gauze pad for a few minutes. Clean, superficial cuts can be dressed with a small adhesive plaster as described in Step 3: Dressing, on page 41.

⊕ Always seek medical attention if:

- the child requires an anti-tetanus booster (*see* Tetanus, page 46);
- the wound gapes and may need stitches;
- there is a lot of dirt or other foreign matter visible in the wound;
- the laceration involves the hand;
- the laceration involves the scalp, an eye or the lips;
- there is a deep laceration on the chest or abdomen.

Left top: Gently clean the graze with a sponge dipped in a diluted antiseptic solution.

Left: Use tweezers to remove any pieces of dirt and grit from the wound.

PUNCTURE WOUNDS

These deserve special mention because of the higher risk of infection, particularly if they occur on the hand. Any domestic tools, cutlery or similar sharp objects that puncture the skin with force may cause considerable damage to the flesh, as well as injecting dirt deep under the skin. These wounds need to be washed out and possibly opened under anaesthetic to ensure all foreign matter is cleaned out.

Puncture wounds on the chest or abdominal wall may have damaged an underlying organ and should always be assessed by a doctor.

➕ FIRST AID Wash the wound under an open tap for two minutes before covering it with a clean dressing. Puncture wounds should be examined by a doctor as soon as possible as they carry a risk of tetanus infection (*see* Tetanus, page 46).

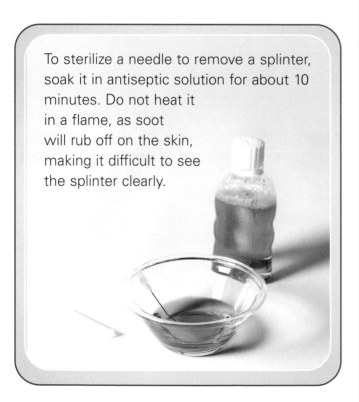

To sterilize a needle to remove a splinter, soak it in antiseptic solution for about 10 minutes. Do not heat it in a flame, as soot will rub off on the skin, making it difficult to see the splinter clearly.

SPLINTERS, FOREIGN OBEJCTS

Thorns or fine splinters of wood, metal or glass can easily become embedded in the soft skin of the soles of little feet, or fingertips. Even the tiniest splinters will sting, particularly if they get into the weight-bearing part of the foot. The discomfort and the risk of infection are two good reasons to do your best to remove the objects.

➕ FIRST AID Only try to remove splinters or foreign bodies you can see. Those projecting outside the surface of the skin can be gripped with a pair of tweezers and pulled out. Wash and clean the skin well afterward with antiseptic solution.

Tiny splinters or thorns that poke out of the skin but are difficult to grip can be removed by wetting the skin and gently rubbing it with a pumice stone. Do not rub back and forth but only in the direction the splinter appears to be pointing.

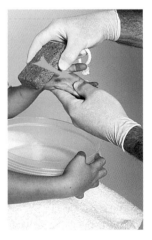

Gently rub in the direction the splinter is pointing.

If the object is completely embedded under the skin, but still visible, soak the area in dilute antiseptic solution for at least 10 minutes to soften the outer layer of skin, making it easier to tease the splinter out. Using a sterilized sewing needle, gently scratch away at the softened skin over the splinter. Once you can grip the end of the splinter with your tweezers, gently pull it out, taking care not to bend or break it. This method is not very painful, but requires the child's cooperation. If she is very anxious, or struggles against you, rather seek medical assistance.

Do not try to remove larger penetrating objects such as twigs, shards of glass or metal fragments which become deeply embedded in the soft tissues. Take the child to hospital immediately, as it may be necessary to take X-rays, or remove the object under a general anaesthetic. Deep penetrating wounds usually require an anti-tetanus booster as well.

BITES

Animal and human bites break the skin, crush underlying tissues and inject saliva, which always contains bacteria. This combination of factors creates a high risk of infection, particularly with bites by rodents, cats and humans, and especially with any bite to the hand.

➕ FIRST AID The key to preventing infection is rapid and thorough cleaning of the wound. Wash the wound as described on page 40. Then cover it with a clean dressing and take the child to a doctor or your nearest hospital immediately. The risk of tetanus and other infections rises with each hour of delay before treatment, so all bites that break the skin must be treated by a doctor without delay. If the wound is a large one, it may have to be cleaned under a general anaesthetic, so do not give the child anything to eat or drink after the injury.

An anti-tetanus booster may be necessary. Antibiotics may be prescribed to combat other bacterial infections, so make sure you tell the doctor if you know your child has an allergy, particularly to penicillin or other drugs.

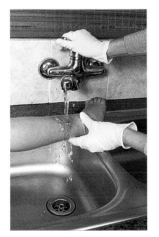

Run tap water over a bite wound to clean it.

Rabies

Bites caused by stray or wild animals, or domestic animals that are acting strangely, might carry a risk of rabies. Make sure to tell the doctor who treats the bite if you have any suspicions about the animal.

Preventing animal bites

Having a domesticated animal for a pet is one of the great joys of childhood. However, make sure your choice of pet is suitable for your child's age, the size of your home and how much time you have to care for the animal. Dogs, cats and domesticated rodents such as rabbits, hamsters and guinea pigs obtained from reputable pet shops or dealers will seldom act aggressively as long as they are disease-free and properly cared for. Dogs, however, particularly larger breeds, need regular exercise, and will become aggressive if kept indoors or restricted to a small garden all day.

Follow these guidelines to decrease the risk of bites and other injuries.

- Some classes and breeds of dogs are more suitable than others for families with small children. To help you make an appropriate choice, seek the advice of a reputable breeder recommended by a kennel club. Ensure pets are vaccinated against common diseases as recommended by your vet or the breeder.
- Unless you have experience in training animals, take your new dog to an obedience class with a professional trainer. Learn to control the dog instead of having him control you.
- All dogs should be neutered, unless bought specifically for breeding purposes.
- Never leave babies or toddlers unsupervised with any animal – even your own pets.
- Consult your veterinary surgeon about any animal that seems to be ill or behaves abnormally.
- A child with a fresh wound on any part of the body should not have physical contact with pets until the wound is properly healed.

- Encourage children to wash their hands after playing with the pet.
- Teach them to keep away from stray animals, and never to provoke dogs – especially those restrained on leads, in cages, or behind fences.

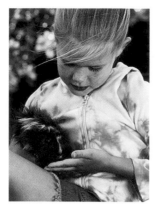

Always wash hands after handling animals.

Tetanus

Tetanus (lockjaw) is a life-threatening infection. The bacterial organism responsible (*Clostridium tetani*) is found in all types of dirt and soil and is particularly widespread in manure and other animal waste. Once it enters the human body through an open wound it targets the spinal cord, releasing a toxin that causes severe muscle spasms and breathing difficulty. Death can occur from heart or lung failure.

Tetanus is very difficult to treat as it does not respond to antibiotics once symptoms appear. Children are routinely immunized against it by standard vaccination schedules (*see* Immunization, pages 142–144.) Wash and clean all open wounds within six hours of injury to reduce the risk of infection.

Your child needs an anti-tetanus booster if:

- he did not get one as part of the routine childhood immunization schedule;
- he has not yet had all his routine childhood immunizations (three doses of the triple vaccine) or you are not sure what he has had so far;
- he is fully immunized, but it has been more than five years since he last had a tetanus booster;
- he has a dirty wound, a puncture or bite wound, a burn wound (*see* Burn Injuries, pages 72–76), or any wound that may be contaminated with manure or other animal waste.

MORE SERIOUS INJURIES

Minor scrapes, cuts and bruises can be adequately and easily dealt with at home. Proper washing, cleaning, and dressing as recommended in these pages will ensure they heal quickly without infection or other complications. However, wounds that carry a high risk of infection or other complications should be examined by a doctor or nurse as soon as possible.

Always seek medical attention for:

- wounds that have not been washed and cleaned within six hours of injury;
- infected wounds – the surrounding skin is red and puffy, and there is a yellowish discharge and increasing pain;
- wounds contaminated with visible dirt, soil or other foreign matter;
- animal or human bites that have broken the skin;
- deep lacerations of the chest or abdominal wall;
- all puncture wounds;
- wounds that need stitches;
- wounds that continue to bleed through the dressing, despite adequate pressure;
- any penetrating wound below the wrist – because of the risk of tendon or nerve injury;
- open wounds involving the lip or the eye;
- any wound associated with painful movement of the underlying bone or joint (*see* Bone and Joint Injuries, pages 47–52);
- scalp wounds associated with symptoms of brain injury (*see* Head and Neck Injuries, pages 53–56);
- any wound that carries a risk of tetanus.

BONE AND JOINT INJURIES

Young, growing bones are more elastic and flexible than those of adults. They often bend rather than snap under force, so fractures are uncommon before a child begins to engage in outdoor activities and games. Fractures before the age of two, repeated fractures, or fractures that occur without significant trauma may be due to an inborn disorder of bone formation (brittle bones). If your child suffers fractures of these kinds, consult an orthopaedic surgeon who specializes in children's diseases.

The bones of the arm and shoulder may fracture when the child falls on an outstretched hand, but the larger bones of the leg require much more force to be broken – the type of impact that occurs in falls from a height or road traffic accidents. Fractures of the hand and foot are mostly caused by crush injuries, as when the hand is caught in a closing door, or something heavy falls on the foot. Injuries to any part of the skeleton may occur in team sports – particularly in contact sports. Joint dislocations are less common in childhood than fractures, and usually occur in association with a fracture.

SPRAINS AND STRAINS

Injuries to the ligaments around joints occur in older children, particularly at the knee and ankle, but usually together with bony injury. The actively growing bones of younger children are more susceptible than the ligaments to injury, and fractures may be missed unless the injured child is carefully assessed by a doctor. Before you decide it is just a sprain or a strain, see the doctor to have X-rays taken so that bone injury can be ruled out.

Depending on the extent and angle of the force applied, a child's bones may fracture completely, or splinter so that part of the bone remains intact (the greenstick fracture). Any force applied along the length of the bone may cause a compression or buckle fracture, where the bone is distorted, but not broken.

Three types of bone fractures

Greenstick fracture
bone bends rather than breaks; minimal damage occurs in surrounding tissue

Simple fracture
bone breaks in one place

Compound fracture
bone sticks through the skin and may damage blood vessels and muscles

GROWTH PLATE INJURIES

Near one end of each bone in the developing child's upper and lower limbs is a growth plate – a soft cartilaginous disc containing specialized cells that produce new bone tissue essential for growth. They continue to produce new bone tissue until the mid to late teens, when circulating hormones cause the growth plate to 'close' and skeletal growth ceases.

Fractures involving the 'open' growth plate are particularly common at the wrist, shoulder, and around the knee. Any swelling and tenderness at those parts of the skeleton should be regarded as a possible growth plate injury until shown otherwise on X-ray.

Failure to diagnose and treat these injuries quickly and correctly may result in permanent damage to the bone-producing cells, and the possibility of abnormal growth, even a complete cessation of growth in that particular bone. The cartilaginous growth plate is the most vulnerable part of the developing skeleton, more prone to injury than even ligaments and tendons. For this reason, 'sprains' and 'strains' are rare in children, and should only be diagnosed by exclusion when X-rays show no evidence of a fracture.

COMPOUND FRACTURES

In severe crush injuries, sharp bone fragments can pierce the skin from inside. Compound fractures carry serious risk of bone infection, which may prevent normal healing unless treated in hospital within six hours.

Nerves and blood vessels near a fracture or dislocation may be compressed by a blood clot that forms around a damaged bone, or lacerated by bone fragments. This is more likely with injuries around the elbow and knee where arteries and nerves lie close to the bone. There is a risk of tetanus infection (*see* Tetanus, page 46) in skin wounds contaminated with soil or dirt.

Signs of bone and joint injury

The four main signs of fracture or dislocation are:

*   pain;
*   swelling caused by bleeding from the damaged bone and muscle;
*   deformity because bone ends are displaced or twisted at an angle;
*   loss of movement – when the child immediately stops moving the affected arm or leg.

Other signs are:

*   punctured or lacerated skin, which together with the signs above may indicate a compound fracture;
*   numbness or pins and needles below the fracture, which may indicate nerve injury;
*   pale, cold skin below the fracture, which may indicate blood vessel injury. Even if you are able to feel arterial pulses below the fracture site, this does not necessarily mean there has been no arterial injury. Check for other signs of poor circulation (*see* The ABC of Life Support, pages 18–27).

Injury, infection or inflammation?

Because healthy children run, bounce and jump through life, our first response to any complaint of pain in an arm or leg is understandably to treat it as minor injury. But, although far less common than injury, acute infection or inflammation of a bone or joint does occur in childhood, and can be very difficult to distinguish from a bump, bruise or fracture. Bacterial infection of bones and joints carries a high risk of spreading to other parts of the body and can lead to chronic infection unless it is treated urgently by an orthopaedic specialist.

Seek medical opinion urgently for any child who complains of limb pain without a clear history of injury, especially if she feels unwell or has a fever.

⊕ FIRST AID A fracture or dislocation may be painful but is seldom life-threatening. If a child sustains severe or multiple injuries from any cause, always focus on the ABCs and provide basic life support if necessary (*see* The ABC of Life Support, pages 18–27) before paying attention to the bone injury. Then proceed as follows:

- Call an ambulance if the child is unable to walk.
- For lower limb injuries, give first aid where the injury happened. Do not move the child unless absolutely necessary.

- Do not move or try to straighten a bent limb as you may do further damage. Instead, leave it in whatever position you found it.
- Cover any skin wounds near the fracture with a clean gauze dressing.
- For crush injuries, apply ice or a cold compress for 15–20 minutes to reduce swelling.
- Immobilize the injured limb by splinting it as shown in the next few pages. This will help to reduce pain and bleeding, as well as the risk of injury to nerves and blood vessels.

SPLINTING FRACTURES BELOW THE ELBOW
(including the hand)

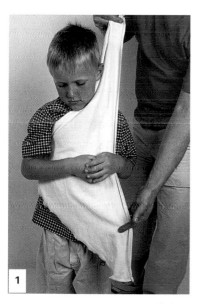
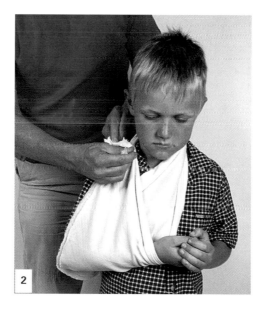
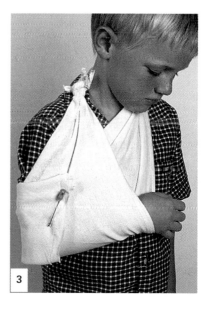

1. Prepare a triangular bandage while the child supports the injured arm.
2. Position the sling so the ends are away from his neck, to reduce movement and minimize keep pain. If the elbow joint itself is injured, do not try to move it. Tie the ends securely so the knot is positioned away from the neck.

3. Always apply the sling to the arm in whichever position you find it. Do not bend the elbow beyond 90 degrees; bone fragments can press on nerves and vessels that run in front of the elbow and may interfere with blood flow. For the same reason, never apply any sling or dressing that encircles the arm tightly at any point.

SPLINTING FRACTURES ABOVE THE ELBOW
(including shoulder and collarbone)

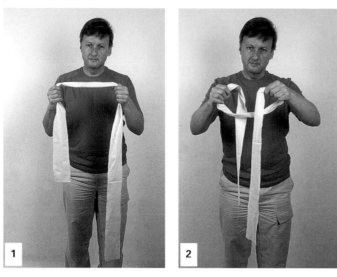

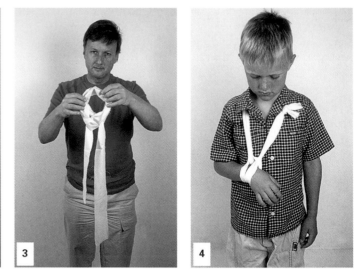

1. Grab a 1m (3ft) length of flannel or linen away from the centre so that you have one long end and one shorter end.
2. Fold two loops as shown.

3. Superimpose the two loops to form a clove hitch.
4. Place the superimposed loops carefully around the wrist of the injured arm and tie the ends securely together.

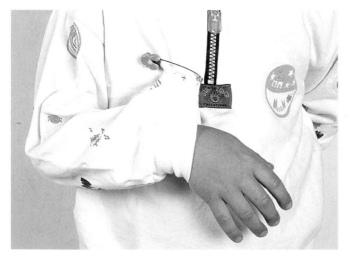

If you do not have a large triangular bandage, you can attach a long sleeve to the front of the child's shirt with a large safety pin. Do not bend the elbow beyond 90 degrees.

SPLINTING A FINGER

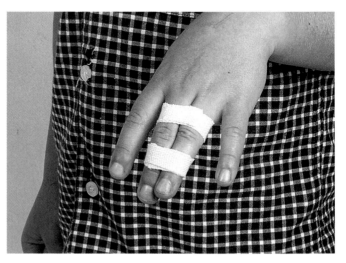

Do not try to straighten a fractured finger, but immobilize the injured finger by strapping it securely to the next finger.

SPLINTING FRACTURES BELOW THE KNEE

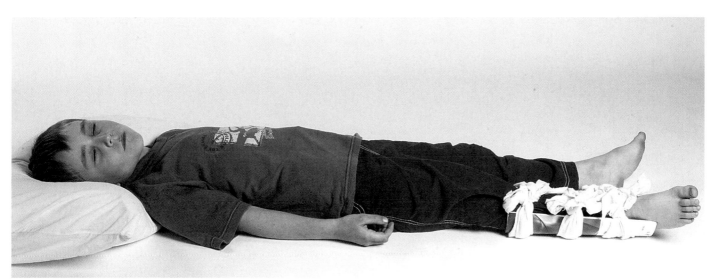

If you have called the ambulance, simply support the calf with a pillow, a rolled-up towel or blanket. If you must transport the child yourself, splint the lower leg with a rolled magazine, newspaper or any sturdy object that extends a few inches above the knee and below the ankle. Foot injuries do not need splinting, particularly if the child is small enough to be carried.

SPLINTING FRACTURES ABOVE THE KNEE

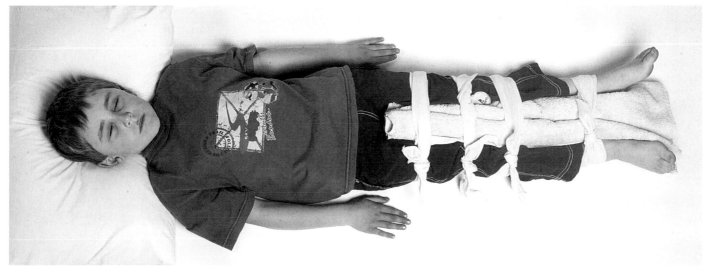

Splint the injured leg to the opposite limb using four 1m (3ft) lengths of linen or adhesive plaster. Do not move the child; wait for the ambulance and allow ambulance staff to move him.

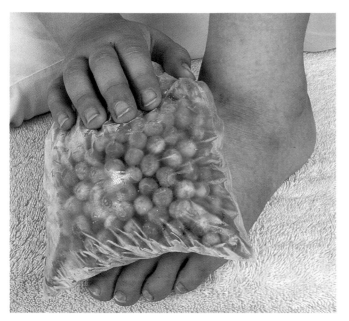

If a child's toes have been crushed, apply a cold compress (or frozen peas) to help reduce bruising and swelling, and take him to the doctor.

Pain relief – Pain at the fracture site is mostly due to the broken bone ends rubbing against each other. This can be minimized by splinting the limb and moving the child as little as possible.

Waiting for the doctor

Do not give a child with a fracture anything to eat or drink before a full medical examination has been done. Until X-rays have been taken, it is seldom possible to know which injuries require resetting under general anaesthetic. Food or drink in the child's stomach may delay treatment.

Aftercare

Most uncomplicated fractures and dislocations that are treated quickly and appropriately should heal completely. Although fracture treatment always attempts the best possible realignment of a broken bone, getting

it perfect is not always possible, or necessary. Slight angles or overlap at the fracture site will often be remoulded as the bone grows in the months after injury. Sometimes metal implants may be necessary to keep the healing bone in an acceptable position.

If the child's fracture is treated with a plaster of Paris cast or splint, ensure that before you leave the hospital you are given precise instructions about looking after the cast. The orthopaedic surgeon will also advise you about how long to restrict the child from sport or other physical activities.

A painful plaster cast

A fracture which has been properly reset and immobilized in a plaster cast may throb a bit, but mild painkillers such as ibuprofen – Brufen™ or Advil™ – or paracetamol (acetaminophen) – Panado™, Calpol™ or Tylenol™– should suffice. Persistent or increasing pain inside a cast requires immediate medical attention to ensure that the blood supply to the limb is not obstructed.

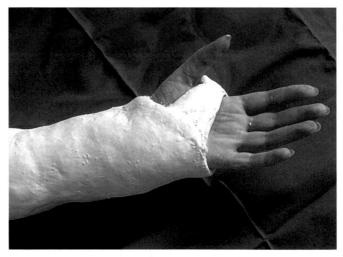

Ensure the plaster cast is not too tight. Any swelling may indicate constriction of the blood flow, so consult your doctor.

HEAD AND NECK INJURIES

Because the brain grows so rapidly in early childhood, a child's head is bigger and heavier in proportion to the rest of the body than that of an adult. By the age of five, the child's brain is almost as heavy as an adult's, although the rest of the body obviously is not. As you would expect, big heads perched on little bodies often get bumped – particularly at the stage when infants are taking their first shaky steps and toddlers are discovering the joys of running, jumping, climbing, and doing everything with more energy than judgement!

KINDS OF HEAD INJURY

Most childhood head injury is 'closed', that is, caused by blunt impact, so that the brain is 'shaken up' inside the skull to a greater or lesser degree, depending on the force of the impact. Penetrating (or 'open') injuries from bullets, knives, stones, and other projectiles are generally far more serious as they can cause severe brain damage.

The brain is well protected by the watery cerebrospinal fluid (CSF), membranes known as the meninges and the skull, which together absorb most of the impact in an injury. Closed head injuries that commonly occur around the home thus seldom damage the structure or substance of the child's brain. However, sudden movement or impact may temporarily disrupt the brain's electrical activity, causing the symptoms that are commonly referred to as concussion.

Cross-section of a skull

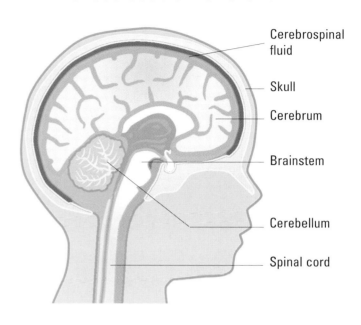

- Cerebrospinal fluid
- Skull
- Cerebrum
- Brainstem
- Cerebellum
- Spinal cord

More severe injury, for example, intentional blows to the head, or falls from a height of several metres, may cause bleeding inside or around the brain, even if the skull is not fractured. Severe, high-velocity impact may also cause the brain to swell so that pressure rises inside the skull. This may interfere with the blood supply to the brain. Brain swelling is an extremely serious complication of severe head injury, but can be minimized by quick and appropriate first aid and basic life-support measures.

The neck can absorb a fair amount of impact without being damaged, as it is protected by the elastic ligaments and discs between the vertebrae. However, the spinal cord may be stretched or damaged even when the spine is not fractured or dislocated.

Fractures of the skull are mostly minor, and will heal without long-term effects. If the X-ray shows a fracture,

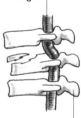

Spinal cord damage

Neck vertebra

this is a good indicator of moderate or severe impact to the brain. Most doctors will want to observe a child with a fractured skull in hospital, however well or unwell the child may be.

A fracture that causes an indentation (a depressed fracture) in the skull may press on the brain and need to be corrected surgically. Some fractures, known as compound skull fractures, may allow CSF to leak out from inside the skull. With these there is a risk of infection (meningitis) and the child may require hospital observation until the leak stops.

Most common skull fracture sites

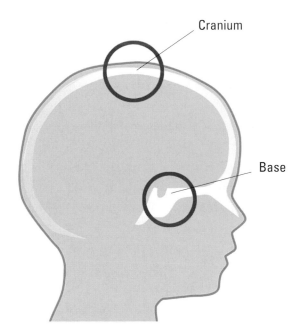

Cranium

Base

Cranial (crown) fractures are usually caused by a direct blow or falling on the head. Fractures of the base of the skull are the result of significant force, such as a road traffic accident or a fall. Raccoon eyes or bruising behind the ear suggest skull base fractures.

Signs and symptoms of head injury

Not all head injury is serious. The vast majority of children who bump their heads will cry lustily, and recover completely within half an hour.

- **The scalp** – You may notice a bruise or small cut at the site of impact.
- **The skull** – Fractures will cause a fairly large accumulation of blood under the scalp soon after injury and the child will inevitably have a headache. Clear or blood-stained fluid leaking out of the nose or ear may be CSF, indicating a compound skull fracture.
- **The neck** – The child may complain of pain or stiffness in the neck. Injury to the spinal cord may cause pins and needles or weakness in the arms or legs. Severe neck injury may cause breathing difficulty owing to paralysis of the diaphragm and chest muscles.
- **The brain** – Mild concussion may cause headache, irritability, nausea and vomiting. The child usually remains fully conscious. If the concussion is severe, however, temporary loss of consciousness and convulsions (fits) are possible, as is nausea. There may be injuries involving the neck and other parts of the body.

Delayed symptoms after head injury

A child may recover quickly after head injury, and then become drowsy or unwell over a period of minutes or hours. This may indicate brain swelling or bleeding around the brain and requires immediate medical attention.

Delayed symptoms – for example, headache, irritability, drowsiness or fever – that only present days after head injury may be due to an unrelated medical condition such as meningitis (*see* Meningitis, page 117). In such cases, consult your doctor as soon as possible.

➕ **FIRST AID** Treat the head and neck as one structure. The child's head is big and heavy, and the neck supporting it is fragile. Imagine an open sunflower on its narrow stem and you will have an idea of what a delicate piece of engineering this is. In response to impact, the momentum of the head inevitably pulls or stretches the neck forward, backward or sideways. This may injure the spine, the spinal cord or both. The more severe the head injury, the more likely the chance of associated neck injury. If your child has suffered a head injury, particularly if he is unconscious, protect his neck carefully until a medical examination and X-rays have shown there has been no damage to the spine or spinal cord.

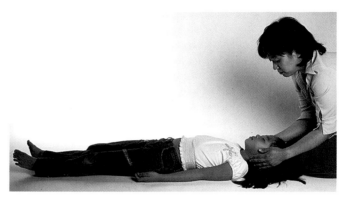

If the child is unconscious, steady the neck to prevent any movement of the spine.

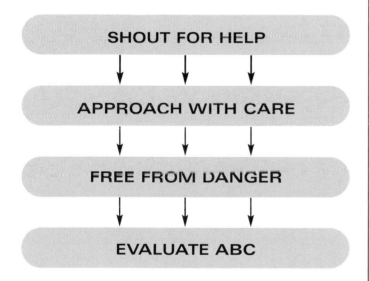

SHOUT FOR HELP

↓ ↓ ↓

APPROACH WITH CARE

↓ ↓ ↓

FREE FROM DANGER

↓ ↓ ↓

EVALUATE ABC

If the child is unconscious or not breathing
- Use the S-A-F-E approach (above).
- Ask someone to call for an ambulance.
- Steady the neck, avoiding any unnecessary movement of the spine.
- Begin basic life support, starting with establishing a clear airway, and continue until help arrives (*see* The ABC of Life Support, pages 18–27).

If the child is conscious
- Press a clean dressing against scalp wounds to stop bleeding (*see* Open Wounds, pages 40–42).
- Treat bruises with a cold compress (ice blocks wrapped in a cloth, or a bag of frozen peas).
- Use a mild painkiller if the child complains of headache.
- Cover the ear with gauze dressing if you see fluid leaking out.
- If the neck is stiffly held in one position, leave it as it is. Support the neck by placing a heavy object on either side until the child is fully awake. Do not force him to straighten a stiff neck, as this may aggravate an underlying injury.
- Keep the child lying down quietly for a few hours. • Watch carefully for any signs of severe injury or deterioration which require medical attention.
- Do not force the child to take anything by mouth. Most children will remain nauseous for at least 30 minutes after head injury and vomit up anything given by mouth.
- Do not plug the ear or nose if you see fluid or blood leaking out.

Seek immediate medical help if:

- the child is not fully awake just after injury;
- he suffers a convulsion after injury, remains irritable or nauseous for more than an hour after injury;
- at first appears well, but becomes drowsy or unresponsive minutes or hours after injury;
- he complains of weakness or numbness affecting the hands, arms or legs;
- he complains of a painful or stiff neck;
- he has a pre-existing nervous system disorder which may make it difficult to assess the effects of injury;
- he has a large scalp swelling suggesting a skull fracture;
- he has clear or blood-stained fluid or blood leaking from the ear or nose;
- pupils are unequal in size;
- he has bruising behind the ear or around the eyes, suggesting a compound skull fracture.

If you suspect the injury or impact to have been severe, whatever the condition of the child, or if you are simply worried, consult the doctor anyway – for your own peace of mind.

Recovery after head injury

Most injuries that do not cause loss of consciousness or structural damage to the brain are followed by full recovery, with no permanent effect on the child's growth or development. He can resume normal activity at his own pace after minor head injury or mild concussion. With more severe injuries that have required hospitalization or surgery, consult the doctor about possible short- and long-term complications. She can advise how soon the child can return to school and resume normal activities. Children who have sustained any degree of injury to the neck may be at risk of re-injury for up to three months afterward. Consult the orthopaedic or neurosurgical specialist who treated the child about when it will be safe for the child to resume sport and other outdoor activities.

Although most children recover quite quickly and completely after head injury, some may be less lucky. Nerve tissue, particularly in the brain, is highly specialized, and once damaged is gone forever, leaving only scar tissue. Ensure your home is safe for children and do your best to prevent head injuries from happening in the first place.

Dealing with suspected skull base fractures

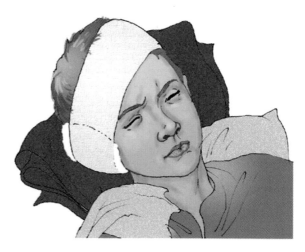

If fluid is leaking out of the ear, use a sterile pad and loose bandage but do not plug the ear.

EYE INJURIES

Of all the special senses, sight is not only the most precious – it is also the most vulnerable. Protect children from severe eye injuries by separating them from potential hazards by as wide a margin as possible – all the time.

- Do not let children of any age play with fireworks.
- Do not let pre-teen children have access to power tools.
- Keep toxic or concentrated chemicals locked up and out of reach.
- Keep firearms locked up in gun safes.

Cross-section of the eye

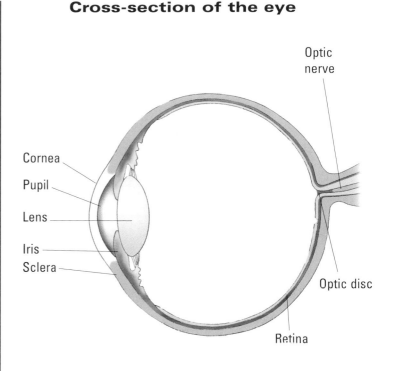

The eye is a highly specialized and delicate organ.

ANATOMY OF THE EYE

The eye is protected by a bony socket, and by the quick shutter-movement of the eyelids, but it is still more exposed than any other special sensory organ.

The eye can easily be damaged by:

- blunt trauma – for example, a punch or a sporting injury;
- sharp objects – for example, a pencil, a pellet from a pellet gun, or a stone thrown up by a lawnmower, foreign bodies, such as dust or sand, or even an eyelash;
- contact with corrosive or toxic chemicals;
- infection, which can complicate any injury that is not quickly or properly treated.

SIGNS OF EYE INJURY

All parts of the eyeball and surrounding tissues are extremely sensitive to any irritation and will show signs of inflammation immediately after any injury. Some of these signs are:

- redness (bloodshot eye) and watering;
- persistent blinking;
- not being able to see clearly;
- a gritty sensation in the eye;
- a bleeding or obviously abnormal-looking eyeball;
- pain (injuries to the cornea are extremely painful).

If both eyes show signs of inflammation, the cause may be an allergy or infection rather than injury. Consult a doctor urgently if you are unsure.

Preventing eye injuries

Although you cannot protect a child from every situation where a piece of grit might get into his eye, you can protect him from severe injuries caused by careless handling of domestic power tools or firearms. These accidents are as unnecessary as they are tragic.

⊕ FIRST AID Since rapid diagnosis and treatment are essential to ensure the best possible recovery from eye injuries, the majority of eye injuries require emergency medical attention from an eye specialist. However, you can usefully apply the following first-aid procedures for foreign bodies in the eye and chemical burns or splashes.

With the exception of these injuries, where first aid can be useful before you seek medical help, all eye injuries should be seen by a doctor immediately.

Foreign bodies in the eye

- Do not let the child rub the eye. This will aggravate inflammation and increase the risk of infection.
- Wait for a minute or two before doing anything. Most foreign objects will be expelled by a combination of blinking and watering. Encourage the child to blink rapidly. If the gritty sensation persists, the object has not been expelled.
- Wash your hands before doing anything further.
- Moisten one end of a clean cotton bud with tap water and have this ready. (A piece of cotton wool moistened and teased into a point will do as well.)
- Gently grip the upper eyelashes and ask the child to look downward as you lift the upper lid forward and upward to get a better view of the eyeball. If you don't spot the foreign object, do the same with the lower lid as the child looks upward.
- If you spot the foreign object lying on the sclera (white part of the eye), dab it very lightly with the moist cotton bud until it comes away.

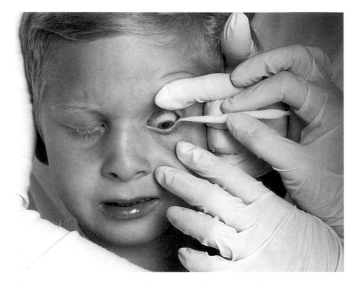

To remove a foreign body, moisten a clean cotton bud or piece of cotton wool. Lift the lid up and get the child to look down.

- Do not persist with trying to remove any foreign matter which seems stuck to the eyeball. What appears to be only a speck may in fact be the tip of a much larger object which has penetrated deep into the eyeball.
- Successful removal will usually bring immediate relief. If the discomfort persists, and you have been unable to spot the foreign object, it may be stuck to the inside of the eyelid. Seek immediate medical attention.
- Do not try to remove foreign objects from the cornea (coloured portion of the eye). Cover the eye (as shown opposite) and take the child to a doctor.
- Do not try to remove foreign bodies if the eye already appears inflamed or infected.
- Do not use rigid or sharp implements to remove foreign bodies.
- Do not struggle with a child who is unable to sit still and co-operate with you.
- Do not put ointments or medications of any sort into the eye unless prescribed by a doctor.

Chemical burns and splashes

Rapidly diluting the chemical with tap water will stop the damage in its tracks. Hold the child's face under a cold running tap and let the water run over the eyeball while you hold the lid open. Continue washing for no less than 20 minutes. You must persist even if the child is uncooperative.

Do not splash water in the eye. This will just make the child blink and prevent water from reaching the eye. Blinking also aggravates corneal damage.

Cover the eye with an eye cup and seek medical attention immediately after washing. Take with you any packaging listing details of the chemical.

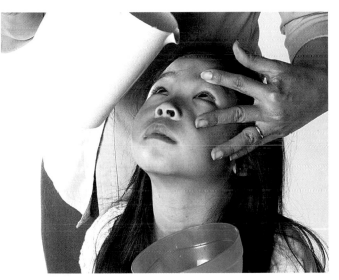

Carefully pour water into the eye to dilute and wash out dangerous chemicals, but do not splash.

Covering the injured eye

The irritated or injured eye is extremely sensitive to light and the child will usually blink continuously. This can aggravate damage that has already been caused to the cornea – that is, the coloured portion of the eye. You can reduce blinking by blocking light from the eye, using the bottom half of a polystyrene cup secured over the eye with a crepe or gauze bandage (*see* First-aid Kits, pages 10–13). Use this method whenever there is even a slight possibility of corneal injury. (For black eye, or peri-orbital haematoma, *see* page 39.)

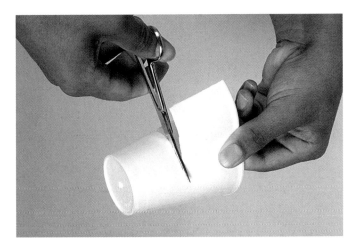

Cut the bottom off a polystyrene cup (above) and attach it with a bandage to protect the eye (below).

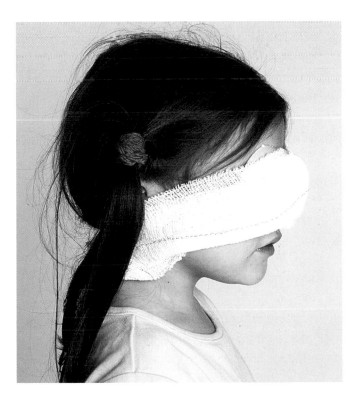

MOUTH, JAW, NOSE AND EAR INJURIES

The tissues of the face, mouth and upper airway are extremely delicate and easily damaged. Impacted foreign objects and lacerations are often self-inflicted, especially in infants and toddlers, who love to stick everything in everywhere. Although most facial injuries tend to be minor, they bleed lustily because of the rich blood supply to this area of the body.

MOUTH INJURIES

Injuries around and inside the mouth are most commonly seen in preschool children, and also in older children who play sport. Sharp objects such as pencils or lollipop sticks carried in the mouth while running may be pushed through any soft part of the mouth if the child falls. A front tooth may be chipped, loosened, or even forced out of its socket if the child falls against a solid surface, or is hit in the mouth with a fist or flying object.

Injuries to the inside of the mouth are dramatic because they are extremely painful and usually bleed a lot. Nevertheless, bleeding usually stops as quickly as it starts, and many of these injuries can be managed at home with a bit of first aid and a lot of reassurance. You can diagnose most injuries with a quick inspection of the open mouth. Use a pocket flashlight to see injuries behind the line of the teeth.

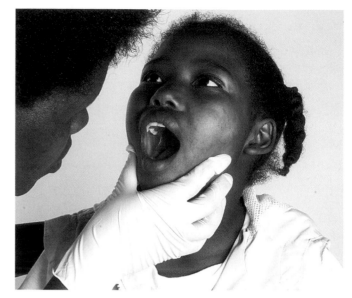

Check inside the mouth to assess the injury.

⊕ FIRST AID For any soft-tissue injury, get the child to lean forward and spit out blood rather than swallow it. You can control bleeding and relieve the pain quickly with a cold compress. Alternatively, get the child to suck an ice cube or rinse out her mouth once with iced water. When the bleeding slows or stops, assess the injury. Small cuts and bites which stop bleeding within minutes will heal quickly, and do not need stitches.

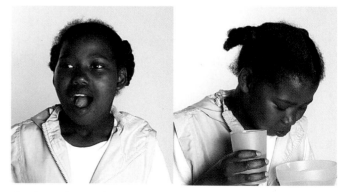

Suck an ice cube to reduce pain, swelling and bleeding or rinse out the mouth with iced water.

Avoid giving the child salty, spicy or acidic foods for five days after injury. Prevent infection with twice-daily tooth-brushing, and rinsing the mouth with water after meals. If gums or teeth have been injured, twice-daily gargling with a mild antiseptic mouthwash can substitute for tooth-brushing for the first few days. Mild bacterial infection sometimes causes injuries to begin bleeding again after two or three days, but good mouth hygiene should prevent this.

Seek medical help if the injury:

- causes difficulty with swallowing or breathing;
- involves the full thickness of the lip, cheek or tongue;
- involves the line where the lip meets the skin or the corner of the mouth;
- creates a large, loose flap of tissue anywhere inside or around the mouth;
- results in bruising or loss of gum tissue around the teeth;
- continues to bleed heavily after a few minutes;
- is at the back of the mouth or throat and difficult to see properly;
- shows signs of infection (bad breath or recurrent bleeding or swelling).

> If your child has orthodontic appliances (braces), the orthodontist or a dental surgeon should assess mouth or dental injuries as soon as possible.

Milk and permanent teeth

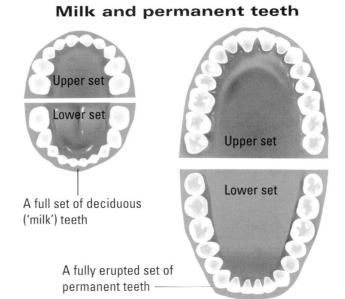

A full set of deciduous ('milk') teeth

A fully erupted set of permanent teeth

Tooth injuries

Just as their first set of teeth is established, children learn to run. Most dentists would probably prefer the sequence to be reversed! Tooth injuries are most common in children aged two to five years, although permanent teeth may also be damaged in older children during contact sports or fights. Front teeth (incisors and canines) are most at risk of injury, and damage to these may be associated with injury to the surrounding gum tissue or the jaw.

FIRST AID All tooth injuries should be assessed by a dental surgeon after you have provided first aid as recommended here. This applies equally to milk teeth and permanent teeth.

Chipped, cracked or broken teeth

- There should be little or no bleeding around the tooth.
- Try not to let the child swallow the loose fragment.
- Larger fragments should be soaked in milk or salt solution and taken along to the dentist.

Loose or displaced teeth

Control bleeding by having the child suck some ice or gargle with cold water. Consult a dentist as soon as possible. Do not try to correct the position of a displaced tooth yourself. This may aggravate bleeding or damage the root.

Lost teeth

Try not to let the child swallow the tooth. Handle the tooth carefully and avoid touching the root. Soak the tooth in milk or salt-water solution. This will prevent the delicate ligaments around the tooth from drying out for up to 30 minutes.

Control bleeding by pressing a gauze swab soaked in cold water against the tooth socket and then take the child and the tooth to a dentist as quickly as possible.

Teeth jammed into the jawbone

Control any bleeding as recommended above and take the child to a dentist as soon as possible.

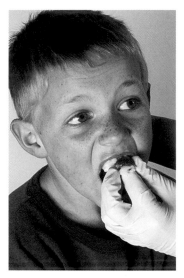

When a tooth falls out, saturate a piece of gauze in cold water and press it into the tooth socket to control the bleeding.

FRACTURES OF THE JAW

It takes a lot of force to fracture the upper or lower jaw. However, suspect this injury if:

- you notice marked swelling or bruising of the gums, in the floor of the mouth or around the lower half of the face;
- he cannot open or close the mouth normally;
- the upper and lower sets of teeth do not meet each other normally;
- two or more teeth appear to be displaced from their normal position.

DENTAL INJURY

The speed with which you respond when your child's teeth are damaged can make all the difference. A dentist may be able to reimplant a permanent tooth which has been knocked out if the root and socket are undamaged. Broken or chipped permanent teeth can be repaired. If a milk tooth is lost, the dentist may use a spacing device to ensure the underlying permanent tooth comes through in the right place at the right time. Even after severe injuries involving several teeth, modern cosmetic dentistry can usually restore normal appearance and function.

Common jaw fracture sites

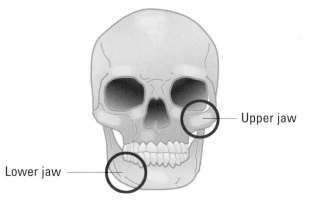

Upper jaw

Lower jaw

Seek urgent medical attention.

Fractures of the jaw require urgent medical attention. Get the child to lean forward and spit out any blood that may be collecting in the mouth. Do not give the child anything to eat or drink, as a general anaesthetic may be needed to reset the jaw, and this may be delayed if she has recently eaten.

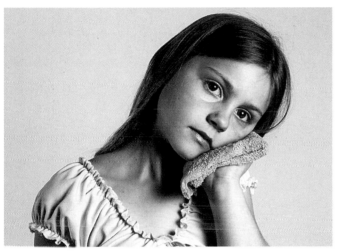

Place a cold compress on the painful side of the jaw and get the child to hospital.

NOSE INJURIES

Although it is a prominent feature on the child's face, the nose seldom lands up in big trouble. The 'bones' of a child's nose are mostly soft, pliable cartilage until they begin to harden with calcium in the early teens, so true fractures of the nose are uncommon in young children. A blow to the nose often causes swelling and some bleeding from one or both nostrils, but it will get better by itself, with little harm done beyond the temporary discomfort and distress at the sight of blood.

 FIRST AID • Control bleeding with direct pressure (*see* The ABC of Life Support, pages 18–27).
- Reduce swelling with a cold compress (ice blocks wrapped in a cloth or frozen peas).
- Use a mild painkiller (acetaminophen or paediatric ibuprofen) for persistent pain.

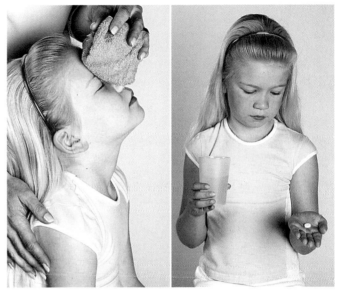

Reduce swelling and bleeding with a cold compress. Give a pill or syrup for persistent pain.

Seek a medical opinion when:

- the nose appears crooked after swelling subsides;
- there is persistent or recurrent bleeding from the nose despite first-aid measures;
- the child cannot breathe through either nostril;
- the outer edge of the nostril has been lacerated;
- there is a foreign body stuck in the nostril (*see* Foreign Bodies in the Nostril, page 70).

INJURIES TO THE EAR

Like the nose, the outer part of the child's ear is mostly soft, flexible cartilage and is therefore fairly resistant to injury. (*See also* Foreign Bodies in the Ear, page 71.)

Bruising of the ear

Blunt impact can cause anything from mild redness and swelling to severe bruising under the skin. The main concern with severe bruising is the pressure that builds up under the skin, which may damage the delicate cartilage. Although rugby players shrug off such injuries, you would probably prefer your child not to develop 'cauliflower ears'!

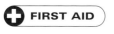 **FIRST AID**

Reduce swelling and bruising by applying a cold compress immediately. Give the child a mild painkiller if needed.

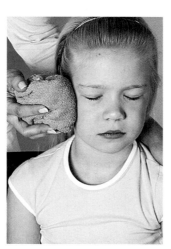

Hold a cold compress against a bruised ear to reduce swelling.

 Seek medical attention if:

- the child complains of severe pain despite having taken medication;
- the skin covering the ear feels tense from built-up pressure;
- there is bleeding from inside the ear;
- the ear appears infected (red, hot and painful);
- the child develops a fever in the days following the injury.

Cross-section of the ear

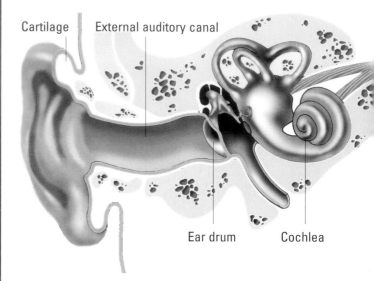

Cartilage   External auditory canal   Ear drum   Cochlea

Lacerations of the ear

Any cut involving the edge of the ear should be treated by a doctor after you have washed and cleaned it. Small nicks and scrapes can be managed at home (*see* Scrapes and Abrasions, page 43).

Bleeding from inside the ear

The eardrum and lining of the ear canal can be damaged by the transmitted force of a firm blow, or the impact of a loud noise or explosion close to the child. She will complain of temporary hearing loss, and there may be bleeding from inside the ear canal.

FIRST AID   Bleeding from inside the ear is usually minimal and stops quickly. If it persists, cover the ear with a few gauze pads kept in place with gauze or crepe bandage. Do not rinse the ear with anything, plug it, or stick anything inside it. A doctor will need to examine the inside of the ear, and may prescribe antibiotics if the eardrum is ruptured.

CHEST AND TRUNK INJURIES

The vital contents of the chest are protected by bone, and severe chest injuries are rare in the home environment. Most injuries sustained by children are cuts, scrapes and bruises of the chest wall, which require nothing more than first-aid attention (*see* Skin and Soft-tissue Injuries, pages 38–43). Where the injury is more serious, however, it is your job to notice the signs and symptoms and ensure the child gets medical attention.

Although a child's ribs are pliable and not as easily broken as an adult's are, a fall from a height or while riding a bicycle may fracture one or more ribs. These injuries are extremely painful, causing agony each time the child breathes deeply or tries to cough. It is usually necessary to admit the child to hospital for a few days.

What you should be most concerned about when your are dealing with a chest injury is the possibility that soft-tissue damage may have gone right through the chest wall – as when a child falls onto a sharp object. This may cause the lung to collapse, or blood may collect around the lung, causing severe breathing problems.

Your role as a first aid provider is to notice the signs that something is wrong with the child's chest, to provide basic life support where necessary (*see* The ABC of Life Support, pages 18–27), and to get the child to hospital as soon as possible.

Anatomy of the upper torso

Sternum

Lungs

Clavicle

Scapula

Rib cage

 Always seek medical attention if:

- the child complains of severe pain when breathing in;
- the child's respiratory rate and heart rate are above the normal range (*see* Tables 1 and 2, page 24);
- the child's complexion becomes pale or dusky (owing to lack of sufficient oxygen);
- one or other side of the chest wall moves abnormally or does not move at all;
- the windpipe just above the breastbone is pushed to one side or the other instead of being central;
- the blood in an open chest wound bubbles each time the child breathes in.

FIRST AID Provide basic life support if the child is unconscious or not breathing. Cover any open chest wound immediately with a clean, thick gauze dressing (two layers at least) fixed in place with short strips of adhesive plaster. Do not worry about cleaning the wound first.

Try to keep the child calm to minimize the body's oxygen requirements. Keep the legs raised above the level of the head if he appears pale or shocked.

Do not bind or strap fractured ribs with bandages; it only makes it harder for him to breathe normally.

Do not probe wounds with your fingers or instruments; this may cause bleeding or introduce infection.

Do not try to remove a sharp object stuck in the chest wall. This should only be done in hospital after X-rays of the chest are taken.

Seek medical attention for sharp objects in the chest wall.

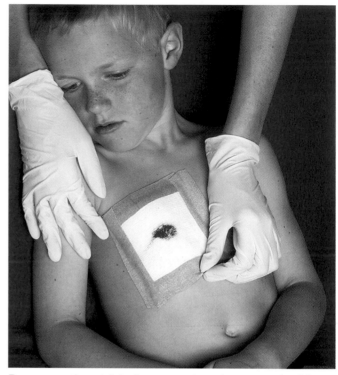

Reassure the child after covering the wound with a clean dressing (above). Keep his feet raised if he is suffering from shock (below).

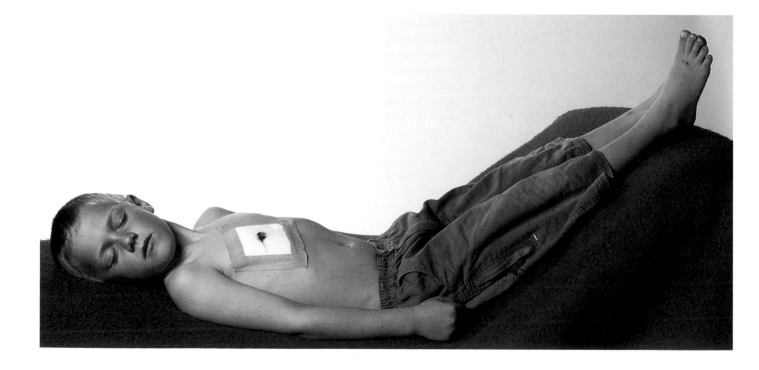

INJURIES TO THE ABDOMEN, PELVIS AND LUMBAR SPINE

The digestive tract and bony structures surrounding it are seldom injured by the activities typically enjoyed by children around the house and garden. However, injuries can be caused by blows or falls from a height, or while riding bicycles. Falls from a height onto an outstretched leg may cause pelvic fractures as well as injury to the leg itself. Smaller children should never be allowed to play in driveways, where they are difficult to see and at risk of being crushed by reversing vehicles. Crush injuries to the chest and abdomen are life-threatening. Your role as a first aid provider is to distinguish as early as possible between minor scrapes and bruises of the body wall, which you can treat yourself, and the possibility of internal injury or fractures, which must be dealt with by the doctor.

Always seek medical attention for:

- deep penetrating injury of the skin and muscle, with or without protrusion of abdominal contents;
- abdominal pain that does not get better or disappear within 30 minutes of injury;
- nausea, vomiting or loss of appetite that does not get better within 30 minutes of injury;
- a child you have witnessed receiving a crush injury to the trunk – for example, the child was driven over by a car;
- pain in the lower abdomen, with difficulty in standing or walking (possible pelvic fracture?);
- a child who complains of numbness or weakness in one or both legs (possible spinal injury?);
- a child who passes blood in the urine minutes or hours after injury;
- a child who appears pale or shocked after injury to the trunk;
- a child whose abdomen becomes swollen.

FIRST AID
- For trunk injuries, if the child is unconscious, appears shocked or has trouble breathing, use the S-A-F-E approach (below).
- Ask someone to call an ambulance immediately. Establish an airway and begin basic life support if necessary. Continue basic life support until help arrives (*see* The ABC of Life Support, pages 18–27).

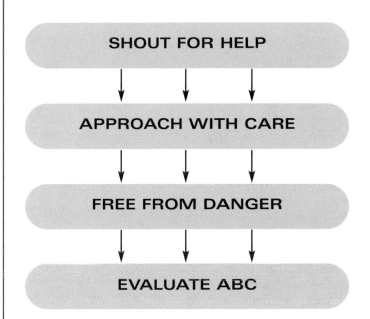

- Do not move a child who is unable to stand or walk.
- Call for help.
- Cover the child with a blanket and raise the legs above the level of the head to improve circulation.
- Cover any penetrating wounds with a clean gauze dressing.
- Seek urgent medical attention for any child with signs of severe trunk injury.
- Do not give a severely injured child anything to eat or drink, because a general anaesthetic may be needed in hospital.

FOREIGN BODIES

The term foreign body refers to any object or material lodged in a part of the body where it does not belong. For example, an item of food that is normally welcome in the child's stomach becomes a foreign body when it is stuck in the ear or inhaled into the lung.

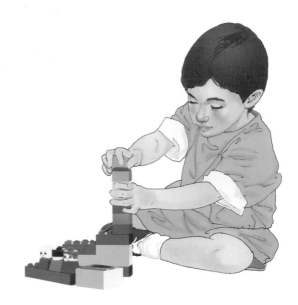

Beware of small toys or toy parts that can easily be swallowed or inhaled by young children.

Foreign bodies are a particular problem in small children, who stick objects into various parts of their anatomy out of curiosity or boredom. They do this with whatever they can lay their hands on, so the list of potential foreign bodies is limitless. Pencils, crayons and sticks may be used to scratch an itchy nose or ear, and then get stuck or break off. The mouth is a favourite place for storing coins or small toy parts when little hands are full, and peanuts and other small food items can go down the airway (the 'wrong way'), particularly when an entire handful is swallowed all at once, or the child is distracted by some other activity.

Objects stuck in the nose or ear may cause discomfort, but they are not a great danger to your child if spotted and removed as soon as possible. However, objects placed in the mouth may be dangerous. A small object such as a peanut or piece of popcorn inhaled into the lung and stuck there can cause chronic infection until the diagnosis is made and the object removed under anaesthetic. And any object stuck in the throat or upper airway may cause breathing difficulty or choking.

Choking on foreign bodies causes approximately 10% of injury-related deaths in small children. Almost all such deaths occur in the home. A combination of home safety measures and adult supervision can significantly reduce the risk of injuries of this kind. (*See* Safety in the Home, pages 31–37. For foreign bodies in the eye, *see* Eye Injuries, page 58.)

SWALLOWED FOREIGN BODIES

You will usually be aware of this problem after seeing it happen or the child is able to tell you about it. Otherwise, suspect a swallowed foreign body if:

- a contented, healthy child suddenly begins to drool or retch;
- the child refuses to eat, or vomits everything taken by mouth;
- any small object with which the child was playing suddenly disappears.

⊕ FIRST AID If the child is choking or has any breathing difficulty, follow these basic guidelines.

- Shout for help.
- Start basic life support.
- Use the 'choking' technique appropriate for the child's age (*see* The Choking Child, pages 28–30).
- Get a medical opinion as soon as possible. The doctor may take X-rays to see if there is a foreign object and if so, where it is, to decide whether an operation is needed to remove it. Objects that have passed into the stomach will usually be left to find their own way out in the stool. Do not use laxatives to speed up the passage of foreign bodies. This only increases the risk of damage to the digestive tract.
- Do not give the child anything to eat or drink, because a general anaesthetic may be necessary to remove the foreign body.

Deliver five firm blows with the heel of your hand between the shoulder blades to dislodge objects.

Foreign bodies in the upper airway

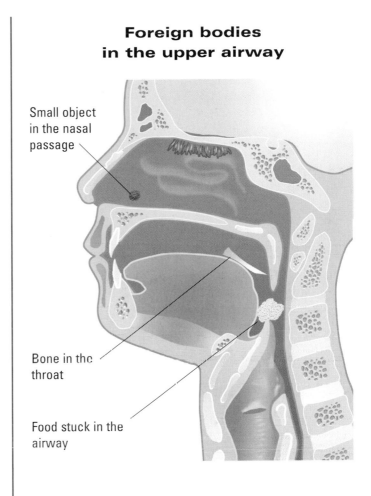

Small object in the nasal passage

Bone in the throat

Food stuck in the airway

Bones in the throat

Small bones from fish or chicken may become stuck at the back of the throat or in the gullet (oesophagus), causing a scratching or burning sensation when the child swallows. These bones often work their way loose if left alone. The discomfort may persist for a short while afterward. If the pain remains severe for more than an hour, get a medical opinion as soon as possible.

Do not try to push the bone out by forcing the child to drink fluids or to eat lumps of bread. The discomfort caused by the bone may make it difficult for the child to swallow normally and he may be liable to choke.

Never stick your finger blindly into the child's throat to try to feel for an obstruction.

FOREIGN BODIES IN THE AIRWAY

Choking may be caused by foreign objects that are too large for the child to swallow and become lodged in the back of the throat. In infants and small children the swallowing reflex is not fully developed, and choking may occur with foreign objects of any size. You should suspect a foreign body in the airway if a child:

- is choking;
- begins to cough, wheeze or struggle to breathe while eating;
- is well but suddenly begins to cough, wheeze, or struggle to breathe;
- develops a persistent cough with fever, which does not get better with antibiotics or other medication.

⊕ FIRST AID If a child is choking or has any breathing difficulty, shout for help and start basic life support, using the 'choking' technique appropriate for the child's age (*see* The Choking Child, pages 28–30).

Even if after first aid the child is able to breathe without too much difficulty, obtain a medical opinion as soon as possible. All foreign objects stuck in the respiratory tract have to be removed.

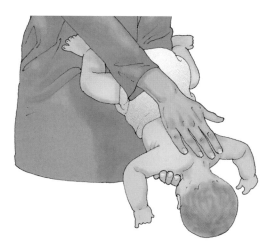

Foreign body obstruction of the airway is a life-threatening emergency.

FOREIGN BODIES IN THE NOSTRIL

You may see the child inserting something up her nose, or the child may tell you about it. Otherwise, you should suspect this problem if:

- she complains of a blocked nose affecting one nostril only;
- she has a foul-smelling discharge or blood coming out of one nostril;
- the skin around one nostril becomes inflamed.

Anything the child can fit into a nostril will be drawn upward with each intake of breath and, because the entrance to the nostril is wider than the deeper part of the nasal passage, it is likely to get stuck at a narrower point higher up. Most foreign bodies impacted in the nose are difficult to see without special lighting or instruments.

⊕ FIRST AID Almost all foreign bodies impacted in the nose must be removed by a doctor. Attempt to remove the object yourself only if it is protruding outside the nostril and can be easily gripped with your fingers. If it does not come away easily, seek medical attention. Do not probe inside the child's nostril with tweezers (or anything else) nor encourage the child to blow his nose. With both manoeuvres there is a major risk of the object dislodging and going into the lung instead.

Successful removal of foreign bodies stuck in the nose or ear requires the child to keep very still. For this reason, many doctors will choose to perform the removal under general anaesthetic. Do not give the child anything to eat or drink before the doctor has decided how best to proceed.

 Seek medical attention for foreign bodies in the nostril.

FOREIGN BODIES IN THE EAR

A small child may try to copy an adult he sees cleaning an ear with a cotton bud or matchstick. Apart from the risk of damaging the delicate eardrum or the skin lining the outer ear canal, this is dangerous as an end may break off and become stuck in the ear. A child with a chronic ear infection or skin irritation inside the ear may use anything long and thin to scratch an itch his fingers cannot reach. Suspect a foreign body in the ear if:

- he keeps complaining of discomfort in one ear;
- he appears to be hard of hearing on one side;
- you notice a smelly discharge or bleeding from one ear;
- the skin of the outer ear has become red and painful from an infected discharge.

✚ FIRST AID Almost all impacted foreign bodies in the ear need to be removed by a doctor. As with foreign bodies in the nose, do not give the child anything to eat or drink before seeing the doctor.

Attempt to remove the object yourself only if it is protruding outside the ear and can be easily gripped with your fingers. If it does not come away easily, seek medical attention instead. Do not probe inside the child's ear with tweezers (or anything else) as this will cause damage to the lining or the eardrum, and risk pushing the object in deeper.

Unwelcome insects

A small insect that flies into a child's ear can cause a lot of distress by buzzing and crawling close to the eardrum.

✚ FIRST AID Warm a small quantity of cooking oil to just above room temperature and pour two drops into the ear canal with an ear dropper. Plug the

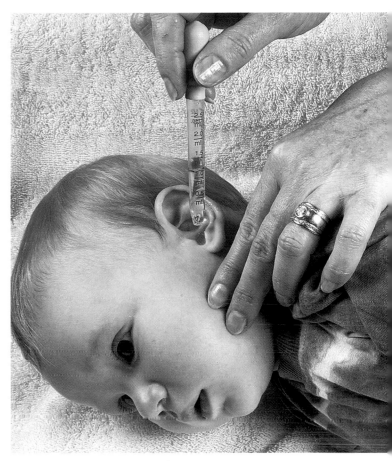

Put two or three drops of tepid cooking oil into the ear to suffocate an insect.

ear loosely with a small wad of cotton wool. The oil will provide immediate relief by suffocating the insect. With the plug still in place, take the child to a doctor to have the dead insect removed.

Foreign bodies in the vagina

This is a problem seldom seen in young children apart from those with mental disability. Foreign bodies in the vaginal opening or canal usually cause irritation and infection within a day or two, and should be suspected in any little girl with groin discomfort, or a vaginal discharge. Only a doctor should attempt to remove a foreign body from the vagina.

INJURIES CAUSED BY HEAT AND COLD

Two kinds of injuries can be caused by extremes of temperature:

- injuries from sunburn, burns and frostbite, which cause local tissue damage;
- injuries from environmental exposure, which cause the body temperature to become excessively high (heatstroke) or low (hypothermia).

Burns are among the most distressing injuries anyone can experience. Even the most minor burns are painful, but severe burns may leave a permanent scar on the child's memory well as on his skin. Children aged two to four years are most vulnerable to burn injuries, but entire families may fall victim to fire caused by faulty electrical circuits, burning cigarettes or leaking gas cylinders.

Only luck determines whether a burn wound will be small or large, superficial or deep. Unlike cuts, scrapes and bruises, which are part and parcel of growing up, burns should simply not happen, and are probably the best reason for taking safety in the home seriously (*see* Safety in the Home, pages 31–37.)

BURN INJURIES

No child should ever have to suffer the agony of a burn injury, and no parent should have to live with the regret of having let it happen. Where burns are concerned, PREVENTION IS EVERYTHING.

Children may be burned by:

- **Hot fluids** – tea, coffee and other hot drinks, boiling water spilled from pots and kettles, bath water that is too hot all cause scalds (*see* Safety in the Home, pages 31–37).
- **Hot oil**, which sticks to the skin, causing a contact injury rather than a scald. Tissue damage is more extensive than that caused by hot water.
- **Exposure to ultraviolet light (sunburn).**
- Contact with **heated surfaces** – pots and pans, stove plates, domestic heaters, even car engines.
- **Chemicals, dry or dissolved in a solution** – swimming-pool chemicals, bleaches and a range of domestic cleaners contain high concentrations of acid, alkali and other corrosive substances that burn on contact.
- **Flame and fire** – apart from burns, there are additional risks of suffocation and lung damage from inhaling hot smoke and poisonous fumes given off by burning chemicals or materials, particularly where children are exposed to fires in confined spaces.

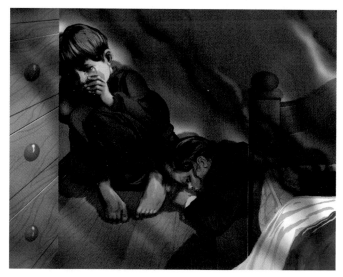

Teach children to lie low in a smoke-filled room to avoid smoke inhalation.

- **Electricity** – skin is a poor conductor of electricity, so it burns at the point of contact with electric current. There may also be a second 'exit' burn at the point where the current leaves the body (*see* Electric Shock, pages 83–84).

Damage from burn injuries is extensive. Heat from any source 'cooks' or 'fries' the skin, and underlying tissues, and the blood in small vessels under the skin may clot, making the damage worse. Serum may leak from the damaged skin and blood vessels, and the larger or deeper the injury the greater will be the risk of shock from loss of fluid.

Remember that any burn injury carries a high risk of infection, and particularly of tetanus (*see* Tetanus, page 46). This is largely because it destroys the skin, which is a natural barrier to harmful bacteria. The amount of tissue damage varies according to heat intensity and duration of exposure. For this reason the first-aid measures described below stress the importance of removing the cause and of cooling the site of injury.

Assessing the severity of a burn

To decide which burns and scalds can be managed at home and which require medical attention, assess the depth of the burn and the size of the surface area affected, using the following guidelines.

The depth

First-degree (superficial)	The skin is red, dry and very painful. The most typical cause is sunburn. Most first-degree burns heal within seven days without scarring.
Second-degree (partial thickness)	The skin is typically blistered and moist, and very painful. These burns may be caused by scalds or fire. They may require skin-grafting. There will be some scarring.
Third-degree (full thickness)	These burns are mostly caused by fire. They involve the deep layers of the skin, which may be pale or charred, and firm and leathery to the touch. Because the nerve endings are usually destroyed, these burns are often painless. All third-degree burns require surgical removal of dead tissue, and skin-grafting. Severe, permanent scarring is inevitable.

The surface area

This may be estimated using the child's hand as a measure. The palm of the child's hand is equivalent to 1% of her Total Body Surface Area (TBSA). As a rule, any burn involving more than 1% TBSA requires medical attention.

➕ FIRST AID Follow these steps, regardless of what has caused the burn or whether the injury requires medical attention.

1. Follow the S-A-F-E approach

SHOUT FOR HELP

↓ ↓ ↓

APPROACH WITH CARE

↓ ↓ ↓

FREE FROM DANGER

↓ ↓ ↓

EVALUATE ABC

Shout for help

For anything more than the most minor burn, ask someone to call an ambulance.

Approach with care

As far as possible, avoid contact with whatever has burned the child. Wear gloves for protection against chemicals.

Free from danger

Remove the child from the source of the injury as quickly as possible. If his clothing is burning, douse the flames with water or smother with a blanket or by rolling him on the ground. Remove outer layers of clothing that are hot or burnt. Take care not to burn yourself in the process.

Evaluate ABC

Open the airway, and check the inside of the mouth for signs of smoke inhalation – redness, swelling, charring, soot particles. Smoke inhalation is life-threatening and requires immediate medical attention. Check breathing and pulse. Begin basic life support if necessary (*see* The ABC of Life Support, pages 18–27).

2. Limit the tissue damage

- Remove tight watches, belts, jewellery or shoes from anywhere close to the burnt skin before swelling or blistering occurs.
- Gently brush dry or powdered chemicals off the skin with a soft cloth before taking the next step.
- Take the container or packaging to hospital with the child, so the doctor can identify the chemical correctly.
- Cool burnt skin under a cool running tap for 20 minutes. Do not use ice or iced water, which will make the skin damage – and the pain – worse. Wash chemical burns for as long as possible but do not delay getting the child to hospital. Wash only the burned area. Do not submerge babies or small children in cold water – this may cause overcooling and hypothermia.

- Gently remove burnt or contaminated clothing that comes away easily, but do not pull at burnt clothing stuck to the skin. Rather use a large pair of scissors to cut around the stuck fabric.

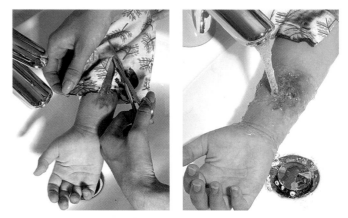

Cut fabric away from the burn site (left) and cool the skin under a running tap for 20 minutes (right).

3. Give pain relief

- The quickest and best relief you can give is to cool the burn. For small burns, acetaminophen (paracetamol) syrup or tablets may be helpful. Burns that are deep or cover large areas of skin will require stronger painkillers which can only be administered in hospital.

Heat remains in a burn wound long after the accident, and goes on destroying tissues until you cool it down. The quicker you can remove the heat source and cool the burnt area, the less tissue destruction and scarring there will be.

- Calamine lotion is soothing for moderate sunburn, but do not use it on blisters, second- or third-degree burns, or on dry peeling skin.

4. Dress and care for the wound

- Cool and cover burn wounds that require medical attention (*see* box on page 76) before taking the child to hospital.
- Use a single layer of kitchen cling film (Glad Wrap™) but remember not to wrap it tightly around a limb; this could cut off the blood supply.

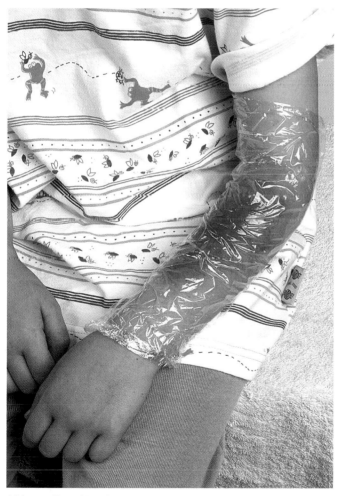

Wrap cling film loosely around a burn wound to seal it from oxygen and stop it from stinging.

- Protect a hand or a foot with a clean plastic bag tied loosely above the wrist or ankle.
- Do not cover the face with anything.
- Large burns may be covered with a clean, dry pillowslip or sheet.
- Do not pop blisters – they may become infected.
- Clean and dress small superficial burns in the same way as abrasions (*see* Scrapes and Abrasions, page 43). Paraffin-impregnated gauze squares are ideal dressings for small burns, and can be kept in place with a gauze bandage.
- Avoid fluffy or sticky dressings, which are very painful to remove.
- Do not put oil, butter, fat or other foodstuffs on a burn wound.
- Do not cover large areas of burnt skin with wet dressings. This may cause a dangerous drop in body temperature, particularly in infants.

5. Promote healing and prevent infection

- Ensure the child gets a tetanus shot (*see* Tetanus, page 46) – even for small burns you treat at home.
- Keep the wound covered with a clean dressing until completely dry. Most minor burns heal within seven days. Change the dressing only if it becomes damp or dirty. The easiest way to remove dressings is to let the child soak in a warm bath.
- Gently discourage your child from picking or scratching at dead skin. This may damage normal skin and delay healing. Reduce the itch by applying plain aqueous cream to the dry or peeling skin. If this does not help, ask your doctor to prescribe a mild antihistamine.

Consider the possibility of infection if:

- there is increasing redness, swelling or discomfort around the wound;
- you notice a nasty smell coming from the dressing;
- you see pus coming out of the burn wound;
- the child develops a fever.

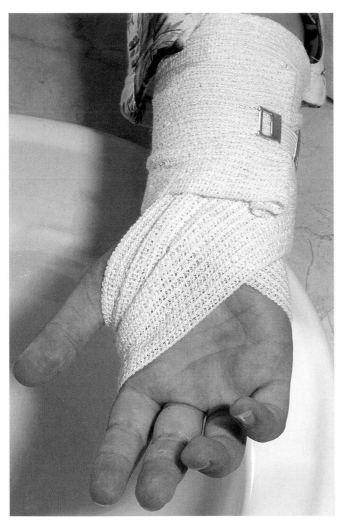

Paraffin-soaked gauze dressings are best for burn wounds. Cover with a clean, dry bandage.

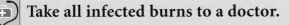 **Take all infected burns to a doctor.**

6. Be aware of some special cases

- Burns to the eye require immediate, prolonged (at least 30 minutes) washing with tap water. If you find this difficult to manage, seek medical assistance immediately. (*See* Chemical Burns and Splashes, page 59.)
- Electrical burns to the skin may be the tip of the iceberg, with much greater damage to the underlying muscle and nerves. Even if the visible burn mark is less than 1% Total Body Surface Area (TBSA), take the child to hospital immediately.
- If the child is caught in a house or room on fire, he may breathe in smoke which burns the airway and lungs, and poisonous fumes from burning materials. Even if there is no sign of external burns, anticipate breathing problems and get the child to hospital immediately.

BURNS REQUIRING URGENT MEDICAL ATTENTION:

- more than 1% TBSA affected;
- all second- and third-degree burns;
- burns affecting the eyes, face, hands, feet or groin area;
- all burn wounds that go all the way around the arm or leg, or a finger or toe;
- all burns caused by chemicals, electricity, fire or explosions;
- all infected burns.

NB: Check whether your child needs a tetanus booster.

FROSTNIP AND FROSTBITE

If a child is exposed to freezing or below-freezing temperatures without adequate protection, ice crystals can form inside the cells of the skin and deeper tissues. Blood may freeze inside small vessels so that the tissues are starved of oxygen, causing permanent tissue damage.

Infants and small children are most susceptible to cold injury, as they cannot control or conserve their body temperature as well as adults, and lose heat quickly. Although these injuries can be extremely painful, children having fun in the snow may be slow to notice what is happening to them.

Cold injury can vary from minor, reversible tissue damage (frostnip) to possible gangrene, with loss of fingertips or toes (frostbite). Damp skin or clothing, wind and prolonged exposure make things worse. Frostnip can usually be treated at home, but frostbite requires urgent medical attention.

✚ FIRST AID for frostnip

Take the child indoors immediately. Remove any wet clothing – gloves, stockings, and so on – and wrap her in a thick, dry blanket. Hold the frostnipped hand or foot in warm water until normal sensation returns. If the water cools, top it up with hot water. Use a cloth dipped in warm water for the face and ears. Give her a hot drink such as tea or cocoa.

✚ FIRST AID for frostbite

Get the child out of the cold immediately. Carry a child whose feet are frostbitten. Call for an ambulance or medical assistance. Remove wet clothes and replace them with warm, dry ones; wrap the child in a thick blanket. Hold the frostbitten hand or foot in warm (not hot) water. Keep it there until help arrives. Use a cloth dipped in warm water for the face. Give a warm drink such as tea or cocoa to restore normal body temperature.

SYMPTOMS OF COLD INJURY

FROSTNIP	FROSTBITE
• Mostly affects the fingertips, toes, cheeks, ears and nose. • The child complains of tingling or experiences numbness. • The affected skin appears red. • Blistering is uncommon. • Usually heals completely within six weeks.	• Commonly affects hands, feet and face, but can affect any part of the body that is not properly insulated against the cold. • Affected parts are numb. • Affected skin may initially appear red, but then becomes cold, white and hard to the touch. • After a while, blisters may form on the skin of the frostbitten area. • Even when treated, frostbite may progress to gangrene, with the affected skin turning black.

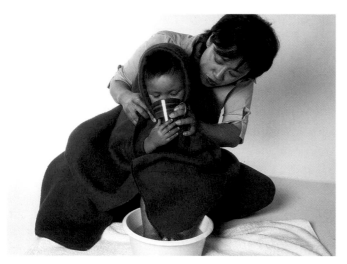

To rewarm a child, put his feet in warm water, wrap him in a blanket and give him a warm drink.

Watch carefully for signs of hypothermia (*see* pages 80–81), which may require vigorous rewarming of the entire body. Do not massage the affected skin or rub it with snow. This will only make the damage worse.

Do not use fires, heaters or hairdryers to rewarm the injured tissue, as this may cause burns. Avoid popping blisters, as this encourages infection.

Preventing cold injury

Before travelling to cold-climate destinations, ask your travel agent or travel clinic for advice on likely weather conditions and recommended clothing. This is particularly important if you plan to take children hiking, or anticipate spending a lot of time outdoors.

Dress children warmly in at least two thick layers of dry clothing before allowing them out into freezing weather. The outermost layer of clothing should be tightly woven and wind-resistant to reduce loss of body heat. Protect the face and hands with scarves, mufflers and mittens or gloves. Protect against dampness with water-resistant shoes and coats.

Clothes or accessories such as scarves should be removed if wet. Replace immediately with dry ones.

If you let children play outside in very cold weather, bring them indoors regularly. Check that all clothing is dry. Give them warm food and drinks, and inspect face and fingers for signs of frostnip. A shivering child should be kept indoors until properly rewarmed.

INJURY FROM EXPOSURE TO HEAT AND COLD

The human body can only function normally within a certain temperature range, and its internal 'thermostat' will maintain that range during brief exposure to excessive heat or cold. With prolonged exposure our ability to regulate body temperature may become exhausted, so that the entire body heats up or cools down too much for organs to function normally. Children are particularly at risk, and they need you to supervise and protect them when they are exposed to extreme heat or cold.

Heat exposure

When it is hot, sweating and changes in blood flow keep the body's temperature constant, and thirst reminds us to replace lost fluid. But although cold water and sports drinks may help to keep the body cool, some children are particularly at risk of overheating. For example:

- infants and small children may overheat after even 20 minutes of exposure to direct sunlight or hot, confined spaces such as a car;
- any child engaging in vigorous exercise;
- a child recovering from recent illness, particularly if he has had fever or diarrhoea.

Symptoms of heat exposure

Illness from heat exposure begins with mild symptoms, and progresses through the four stages shown below. The best thing you can do is protect the child from exposure; your next priority is to notice the problem early, cool her down, and replace fluid in good time.

➕ FIRST AID for heat exposure

Dehydration

The symptoms are thirst, flushed skin and dry mouth, tiredness, headaches, and dizziness. Move the child out of the sun and provide cool drinks. Only allow her back into the sun when all symptoms have completely disappeared.

Heat cramps

Symptoms are muscle pain or cramps during exercise under hot conditions, and possible signs of dehydration. Give the child water or, preferably, a sports drink to replace fluid and essential salts. Gentle stretching or massaging the affected limb may also help. Wait until the pain has completely gone before allowing the child to resume activity.

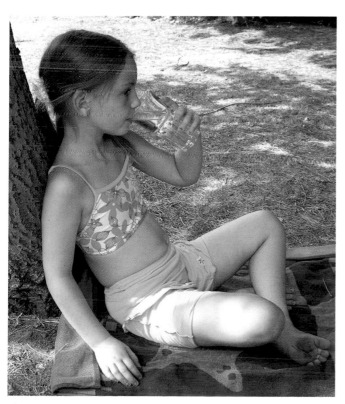

Get the child out of the hot sun, into the shade before doing anything else.

FLUID REPLACEMENT

Whether you are preventing or treating dehydration, cooled sports drinks that contain the correct balance of salt and sugar – and even plain water – are the best options. Avoid sweet, fizzy cold drinks or sodas, which have a high sugar content. The sugar acts like a sponge, drawing water out of the body via the kidneys, aggravating dehydration.

Heat exhaustion

In addition to the symptoms listed above, the child looks pale, sweaty and unwell, and may complain of stomach cramps, nausea, or feeling faint.

Move him to the coolest place available. Remove hot clothing and sponge the body with cool water. Encourage him to drink as much as possible. Obtain medical assistance if he does not recover rapidly, or shows signs of heatstroke.

Heatstroke

The symptoms are as for heat exhaustion, but the child's skin is very hot and dry and he may be drowsy and confused. His heart rate and breathing are rapid. He may vomit or have a convulsion.

Heatstroke requires urgent medical attention. While you wait for the doctor, remove all hot clothing and begin cooling the child down in a tub of cool – but not cold – water.

Alternatively, use wet towels, or a fan, even water from a hose if one is handy.

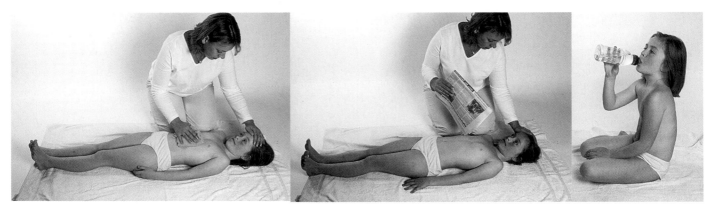

Sponge the child with a damp cloth and fan her skin to cool her down. Make sure she gets plenty fluids.

Preventing sunburn and heat exposure

During hot weather, schedule outdoor activities, outings to the beach, and outdoor games for the morning or late afternoon. Children should stay out of the midday sun (11:00–14:00).

Keep infants out of the direct sun entirely, as they can become dehydrated and sunburnt within minutes.

Following fever or any acute illness, children easily become dehydrated in hot weather and should return to normal outdoor activity gradually.

Protect children against UV light with lightweight clothing and hats. Apply sunblock or high factor sunscreen on all exposed skin. Always reapply after swimming. Consult your pharmacist or family doctor about which sun protection factor (SPF) preparation your child needs. Remember, swimming pools and seawater may keep a child cool, but skin under the water is still exposed to sunlight and must be protected with water-resistant sunscreen. Pack sunblock and sunscreen for holidays in the snow. As long as the sun is shining, sunburn can occur – even in icy conditions.

Encourage children to drink plenty fluids (ideally plain water) during hot weather, especially if exposed to direct sunlight, or playing outdoor sports. Do not wait for them to complain of thirst.

Remember, sunburn may occur together with heat dehydration, heat cramps, heat exhaustion or heatstroke if the child has been exposed to direct sunlight.

Hypothermia

In freezing or near-freezing temperatures, children may lose body heat more quickly than they can generate it. When this happens, their body temperature drops below the normal range. Hypothermia is a very serious condition that occurs when body temperature drops below 35.5°C or 96°F. As the body cools, the brain, heart and kidneys begin to malfunction, and the body will literally freeze unless rewarming occurs in good time.

Babies and small children are as ill-equipped to deal with extreme cold as with extreme heat. In cold climates, babies and infants can become hypothermic while sleeping in an unheated room. The process will be hastened if their clothing or bedding is damp.

The effects of hypothermia

37°C / 98.6°F Normal body temperature

35°C / 95°F

Hypothermia develops

30°C / 86°F

25°C / 77°F — Irreversible hypothermia

20°C / 68°F

A child who accidentally falls into very cold or freezing water may have to be treated for hypothermia as well as near-drowning (*see* pages 96–99).

Signs of mild hypothermia

- The skin is cold to your touch, and has a pale or bluish appearance, particularly on lips and fingertips.
- The child is shivering (a reflex that generates body heat).
- An older child may be lethargic, with poor coordination, even for simple tasks.

⊕ FIRST AID • Move the child to the warmest possible place indoors. If necessary, raise the indoor temperature using a heater or fire.

- Remove and replace any wet clothing, or wrap the child in thick, woollen blankets. Placing the child in a warm (not hot) bath may also help to restore warmth.
- Give the child plenty hot, sweet fluids to drink.
- Check for signs of frostnip and frostbite, and treat as recommended on page 77.

Signs of severe hypothermia

- The body is very cold, almost freezing, to the touch.
- Shivering may be prolonged and impossible to control.

- The skin of the face and hands appears blue or purple.
- The arterial pulse may be irregular, and can be difficult to detect.
- Breathing may become shallow, irregular, or even stop completely.
- The muscles become rigid and feel hard when you touch them.
- The child becomes very drowsy and may be difficult to rouse.

⊕ FIRST AID • First, get yourself and the child out of the cold.

- Reduce heat loss as for mild hypothermia.
- Use your own body heat and skin contact to rewarm infants.
- Commence basic life support if necessary, and continue until normal circulation and breathing are restored, or until the child is rewarmed (*see* The ABC of Life Support, pages 18–27).
- Get the child to hospital or the closest medical help urgently, and continue to administer basic life support en route.

Severe hypothermia is life threatening and requires emergency medical care.

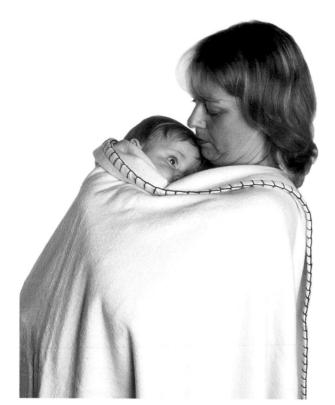

Use your own body heat and a warm blanket to rewarm an infant.

INFANTS AND THE COLD

Infants cannot tell you how cold they are. They do not even know they are freezing. They will cry for a while, as they do for all sorts of reasons. As they become exhausted from the combined effort of crying and trying to stay warm, they will go quiet and lie still. If left alone, without the necessary precautions during very cold conditions, they will freeze and die – quickly and quietly.

Should you check the child's temperature?

Accurate measurement of subnormal body temperature must be done via the rectum, for which you need a special low-reading thermometer. Leave this to the doctor. If your child shows any signs of hypothermia, taking her temperature is simply a waste of time. Do not delay first aid.

Preventing hypothermia (*see* Preventing Cold Injury, page 78)

Infants in cold climates

Where it is difficult to keep the indoor temperature warm during cold conditions, keep infants warm at night by letting them share the bed with you. Take precautions, however, to ensure that you do not roll over and suffocate the infant.

Ways of producing heat

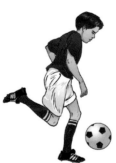

Physical activity

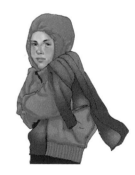

Warm clothing

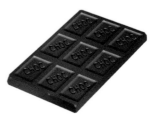

High-energy food

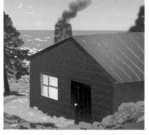

Heated shelter

ELECTRIC SHOCK

Most injuries caused by electricity occur in the home – from contact with electric appliances, power points, faulty wiring, or electricity conducted through water. Infants and toddlers are particularly at risk because they insist on exploring everything with fingers and mouths. Home electrical safety measures should focus on keeping any source of electrical current well insulated and preferably out of their reach (*see* Electrical Safety, page 33).

Because electricity supplied to your home is stepped down from high to low voltage, most domestic electric shocks are minor, causing only a brief, unpleasant 'buzz' and a scare before the child lets go. However, electrical current (particularly alternating current) can also cause muscles to contract involuntarily, so the child cannot let go of the source, which results in more sustained and extensive injury.

The electricity cables that supply our homes carry high-voltage current. Contact with these cables is almost always fatal. Do not let your children play on building sites or near road works where live cables may be exposed.

Depending on the kind of current and how long the contact lasts, electric shock may cause:
- interruption of normal heartbeat and cardiac arrest (heart failure);
- paralysis of breathing;

- damage to the brain and loss of consciousness;
- burn injury at the point of contact and where the current exits the body;
- 'cooking' of nerves and tendons, which conduct electricity better than other tissues; and
- muscle spasms, which may cause the body to jerk, resulting in fractures and dislocations of the spine and other parts of the skeleton, as well as internal injury.

SIGNS OF ELECTRICAL SHOCK

The diagnosis of electric shock is usually obvious when it happens in the home. However, if the injury occurs in your absence, the discovery of a distressed, immobile or unconscious child lying not far from an electrical appliance or power supply should make you suspect electrocution.

✚ FIRST AID 1. The S-A-F-E approach

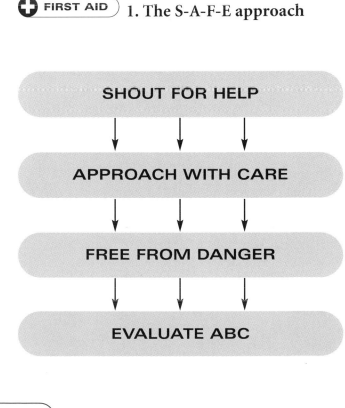

SHOUT FOR HELP

APPROACH WITH CARE

FREE FROM DANGER

EVALUATE ABC

- **Shout for help**
  If the child is unconscious or breathing abnormally, ask someone to call an ambulance immediately.

- **Approach with care**
  Protect yourself from the electricity. If there is water, electric wiring or any other electricity source near the child, you must regard the child as 'electrified', and a danger to yourself.
  Insulate yourself. Water may conduct electricity from the source or from the child to you. Do not approach the child across a wet floor if you are barefoot. Wear rubber gloves and shoes or stand on anything made from non-conducting material (clothing, paper, wood, plastic or rubber) before going near the child.
  Do not go near a child who is in contact with high-voltage electricity cables; call emergency services.

- **Free from danger**
  Unplug or switch off the electricity source only if you can do so without endangering yourself. If not, switch off the main supply at the switchboard.
  Push or pull the child away from the source of electricity, but do not allow your skin to touch his skin. Use a broomstick, chair or any dry, non-conducting object to move him, or simply pull on his clothes.
  No manner of insulation will protect you from high-voltage electrical cables. Stay away!

- **Evaluate ABC**
  If the child is unconscious, check the Airway, Breathing and Circulation. Begin basic life support if necessary (*see* The ABC of Life Support, pages 18–27). Continue until help arrives.

2. Consider other injuries

Keep the child lying still on his back or in the recovery position until help arrives. Unnecessary movement may make a neck fracture or other injuries worse.

3. Check for burns

Remember that there may be skin burns at the sites where current entered and exited the body (*see* Burn Injuries, pages 72–76).

 Call a doctor or take the child to hospital if he has:

- electrical burns involving the hand or mouth;
- infected burn wounds (red, weeping, painful);
- muscle pains or spasms;
- a cough or any difficulty breathing; or
- palpitations (irregular heartbeat).

Do not touch the child; use a broom (far left) or non-conductive material such as a towel (below) to push or pull him away from the source of electricity

POISONING

Serious cases of childhood poisoning most commonly result when toxic substances are taken by mouth or inhaled in gaseous form. Volatile liquids such as paraffin (kerosene), solvents, household cleaning agents or aerosol sprays can cause poisoning by both of these routes. Poisons may also cause local damage through contact with the skin or the eyes.

A s is the case in most childhood injuries, it is the two- to four-year-old age group that is most at risk of accidental poisoning. To a small child, paraffin (kerosene) stored in a lemonade bottle is lemonade, and sugar-coated prescription tablets or vitamins are sweets (candy). Although an older child will spit out anything that tastes revolting, the gagging reflex in infants and toddlers is not fully developed and they will inevitably swallow a certain amount of any poison they taste.

The combination of curiosity, perpetual craving for food and drink, and inability to read and tell one substance from another places toddlers at risk wherever and whenever they have half a chance to access toxic substances anywhere in the home. The key to protecting your child from poisons is to reduce that half a chance to zero. This is best achieved by a combination of adult supervision and blocking access through childproof packaging, and keeping poisonous substances well out of reach – preferably under lock and key.

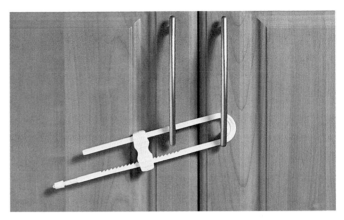

Keep harmful substances in a locked cupboard.

WHERE POISONS LURK

Since the substances responsible for most childhood poisoning are found in the bathroom, master bedroom, kitchen and tool shed or other DIY area, target these sites for poison safety (*see* Safety in the Home, pages 31–37).

The incidence of childhood poisoning from aspirin and other medications has dropped significantly in countries where the law requires them to be dispensed in child-resistant containers. However, even this does not guarantee safety: 20% of preschool children can open them. Constant adult supervision remains the most important child safety measure.

SWALLOWED POISONS

Poisons taken by mouth may make the child ill within minutes by being absorbed through the gut into the bloodstream, and may cause damage to the lining of the digestive tract itself. The toxic effects will depend on the nature of the poison, how much is swallowed, and how quickly it is passed out of the stomach.

Acid (used in swimming pools) and strong alkalis (such as domestic cleaners or bleach) are extremely corrosive; swallowing even small amounts can cause immediate, permanent damage to the delicate lining of the child's oesophagus.

Signs of swallowed poison

Consider the possibility of swallowed poison if your otherwise healthy child suddenly appears unwell, begins to gag or vomit repeatedly, complains of tummy-ache or moves or behaves abnormally.

Some poisonous substances, such as potassium permanganate, can be identified by their smell or a telltale stain on the child's lips and face.

Where the poison has affected the nervous system (for example, painkillers, sleeping tablets or alcohol), the child may be drowsy, difficult to rouse, or deeply unconscious. Finding an open or empty container near the child should help to clinch the diagnosis.

➕ **FIRST AID**   Call your local or national Poisons Control Centre or Helpline. (Ensure the Centre's phone number is clearly marked on the lid of your first-aid kit, and next to each telephone in your house. For good measure, ensure that the number is next to your neighbour's telephone as well.) If you do not have access to a Poisons Centre, get advice from your doctor or local hospital emergency unit.

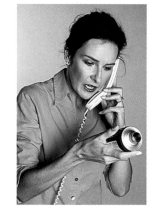

Give any package information to the poisons centre for speedy advice on what to do.

If the child is unconscious or having trouble breathing, use the S-A-F-E approach

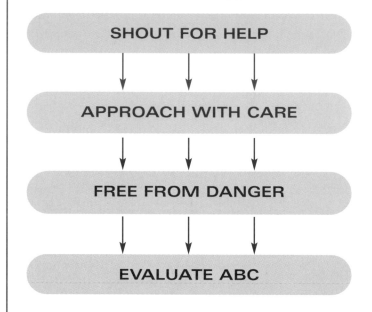

SHOUT FOR HELP

APPROACH WITH CARE

FREE FROM DANGER

EVALUATE ABC

- **S**hout for help. Ask someone to call an ambulance, and then contact the local Poisons Control Centre or Helpline.
- **A**pproach with care. Beware of spilt liquid near the child that may be dangerous to yourself.
- **F**ree from danger. Get the child away from any toxic substance that may be a danger to either of you.
- **E**valuate ABC. Open the airway. Clear away any unswallowed tablets or other poison which you can see in the mouth. Begin basic life support and continue until help arrives.

If the child is conscious
- Get her to spit out any poison left in her mouth.
- Give her half a glass of milk or water to drink. This dilutes poison already in the stomach and limits corrosive damage from acids or alkalis.
- Nurse a drowsy child in the recovery position (*see also* page 23) to protect the airway if she vomits, which is likely.

- Call your Poisons Centre or doctor for advice. Have available the following information:
  - the age and approximate weight of the child;
  - the approximate length of time since the poison was taken;
  - the details of the poison (check the packaging), and how much was taken;
  - any abnormal physical signs you have noticed.
- Follow the advice you are given and take the child to hospital if necessary.
- Do not try to make the child vomit, either by giving a remedy to induce vomiting or sticking your finger down the throat. This is of no benefit whatsoever, and can do significant damage if the vomited poison is inhaled into the lungs.

INHALED POISONS

The common hazards found in the home are:
- leaking gas from a faulty gas supply pipe or canisters used for cooking and heating;
- carbon monoxide that accumulates when open fires are allowed to burn in poorly ventilated indoor spaces;

IPECAC NOT RECOMMENDED

Syrup of Ipecac induces vomiting, and was recommended for many years as a first-aid measure and an essential item in all home first-aid kits. In 2003, however, it was established that administering Ipecac or inducing vomiting by any means is of no benefit in most poisoning cases, as it eliminates very little of the poison already in the stomach. Some children will vomit repeatedly after being given Ipecac. As this may interfere with other treatments they need to be given in hospital, we do not recommend that Ipecac is used in the home.

- flammable materials that catch fire, releasing toxic gases which are breathed in together with smoke (*see* Burn Injuries, pages 72–76).

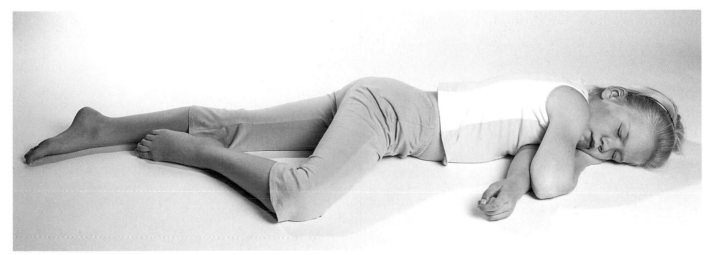

Place the child in the recovery position to ensure the airway remains open in case she vomits.

Intentional poisoning is rare before children reach their teens. Poisons most commonly taken intentionally by adolescents are alcohol, prescription medication and so-called recreational drugs. Teenagers requiring prescribed medication for behavioural or psychiatric disorders should be given only short-term supplies, to reduce the temptation to overdose intentionally. If an older child has harmed himself deliberately, seek medical advice for the underlying emotional or psychological disorder as soon as the effects of the poison itself have been dealt with.

SHOUT FOR HELP

↓ ↓ ↓

APPROACH WITH CARE

↓ ↓ ↓

FREE FROM DANGER

↓ ↓ ↓

EVALUATE ABC

Sadly, the most common poison inhaled by children is cigarette smoke exhaled by their own family members and other adults. While passive smoking may not cause any sudden crisis, it has negative long-term effects on the health, growth and development of your child. Keep your home and your children smoke-free.

The signs of toxic inhalation are usually obvious – particularly in the event of a fire. In fact, if you are alert, you may smell leaking gas even before you come across a child in distress.

If the child swallows a volatile liquid (for example, paint stripper, turpentine or paraffin, or the contents of an aerosol can), it can give off fumes that are inhaled into the lungs as well – two kinds of poisoning in one.

✚ FIRST AID
- Use the S-A-F-E approach.
- Ask someone to call an ambulance.
- Think twice before putting your own life at risk.
- Get the child out of an enclosed space containing toxic fumes.
- Begin basic life support if required. Continue until help arrives.

If the child is conscious and breathing normally, and there is no risk of fire or other danger to your family, it is still a good idea to call your local Poisons Centre or hospital emergency unit for advice. Have the necessary information about your child and the likely poison available when you call.

Contact poisons: Treat as for chemical burns – *see* Burn Injuries, pages 72–76.
Poison in the eye: *see* Eye Injuries – Chemical Burns and Splashes, page 59.

VENOMOUS BITES AND STINGS

With some animal-inflicted injuries the risk of poisoning is of more concern than the damage caused by the bite. Non-venomous insect bites are usually harmless, causing only local discomfort, itching and swelling, but the venom injected by insect stings and the bites of certain snakes and spiders may cause a systemic reaction (one affecting the whole body), sometimes requiring basic life support and a dose of anti-venom.

A poisonous bite or sting may cause an unusually severe reaction in some children who are allergic to the venom, and such children should be protected as far as possible from exposure to this type of injury. During warm weather and when camping or hiking in open countryside, you can avoid stings and bites by wearing protective clothing in neutral colours and closed shoes, and spraying with insect repellents (diethyl toluamide or DEET), particularly if you are out of doors at dawn and dusk – mealtimes for insects. Scented cosmetics and brightly coloured clothes both attract insects, and should be avoided.

(For treating bites by dogs, cats and other animals *see* Bites, pages 45–46.)

✚ FIRST AID   If your child has a severe allergic reaction to a bite or sting, such as an itchy rash with swelling, and difficulty in breathing:

1. Use the S-A-F-E approach (avoid getting bitten or stung yourself).

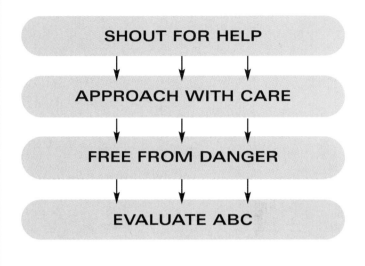

SHOUT FOR HELP

↓   ↓   ↓

APPROACH WITH CARE

↓   ↓   ↓

FREE FROM DANGER

↓   ↓   ↓

EVALUATE ABC

2. Start basic life support (ABC).
3. Open the child's airway.
4. Check for breathing and circulation. If absent or doubtful – continue until help arrives (*see* The ABC of Life Support, pages 18–27).

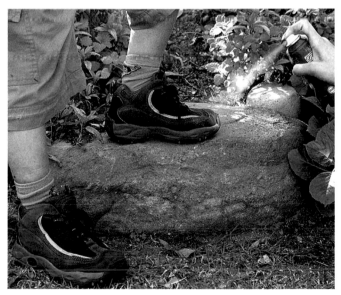

Before a hike in the bush, spray the child's shoes with insecticide to prevent tick bites.

Snake bite

- Never apply a tourniquet!
- Never cut the wound and try to suck venom out 'cowboy'-style.
- A bite or sting that becomes more red, swollen or painful three to five days after injury may be infected. Take the child to the doctor if she seems generally unwell following a bite or sting.

Anti-venom

Specific anti-venoms exist for a variety of venomous creatures. However, we do not advise that you carry these in your first-aid kit unless you have been trained in how and when to administer them. Even then, use them only when you can identify the creature beyond any doubt. Incorrect use of an anti-venom may do more harm than good.

Emergency drugs

If your child is known to be allergic to certain insect bites or stings, your doctor may advise you to keep a pre-packed adrenaline pen or syringe handy at home or in your first-aid kit. Given into the thigh muscle, this drug may be life-saving in the event of severe allergic or anaphylactic reaction (*see* page 107), but must be given correctly. Follow the manufacturer's instructions and – most importantly – your doctor's advice about using it.

FLYING INSECTS

Bees, wasps, hornets and yellow jackets

Flying insects sting anything or anyone who disturbs them or comes near their nests or hives. Honey bees die after stinging, but hornets and wasps can sting again and again.

Children should be warned that even dead insects can sting. In addition, beware of stinging insects floating in your swimming pool.

Symptoms

The sting of a flying insect usually causes a painful red swelling, which gets better within 24 hours. These are dangerous only if there are multiple stings and a large amount of venom is injected, which may cause toxic reactions such as fever, vomiting and malfunction of the kidneys – or if the child is allergic to the venom which can lead to severe allergic reaction.

⊕ FIRST AID Honey bees leave a barb or 'stinger' in the skin. This looks like a small dark splinter in the centre of the sting site, and is attached to a poison sac. Scrape the stinger out gently, using your fingernail, a blunt knife or a credit card. Do not use tweezers – there is a chance you may squeeze additional poison into the child. Relieve pain by applying an ice block or cold compress to the sting area for about 10 minutes. Creams or gel containing the local anaesthetic benzocaine may soothe the sting. Alternatively, try gently rubbing meat tenderizer or baking soda onto the skin around the sting.

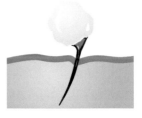

The barb of a bee sting

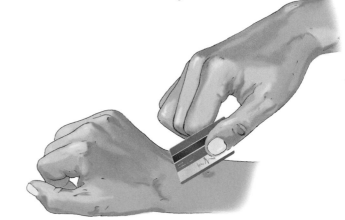

Use a credit card to scrape off the sting; tweezers can make extra poison enter the skin.

Seek urgent medical attention if:

- there is marked swelling, or if it persists for more than 24 hours;
- the child has an urticarial rash (*see* Urticaria, page 139) or facial swelling;
- the child has breathing or swallowing difficulties;
- there are more than 10 stings;
- there is a sting inside the mouth; or
- the child feels unwell after the sting.

CRAWLING INSECTS

Spiders

Only a small fraction of the huge number of spider species is poisonous and only the female bites. The most dangerous spiders are: the **brown spider** (also known as the brown recluse or violin spider), which is widely distributed in warmer countries; the **American black widow**; the **South African button spider**; and the **Australian funnel web spider**

Signs of spider bites

The bite of the brown spider can cause local pain, swelling and a large sore that heals slowly. The black widow, button and funnel web spiders inject venom that attacks the nervous system, causing severe muscle paralysis and breathing difficulty.

 FIRST AID Apply ice or a cold compress to the bite area. Seek urgent medical help for a child who develops any symptoms after a spider bite, especially if you cannot identify the spider. Symptoms of severe poisoning may be mild at first, then become life-threatening within minutes or hours. The smaller the child, the greater the risk of fatal poisoning. If possible, take the dead spider to the hospital to be identified.

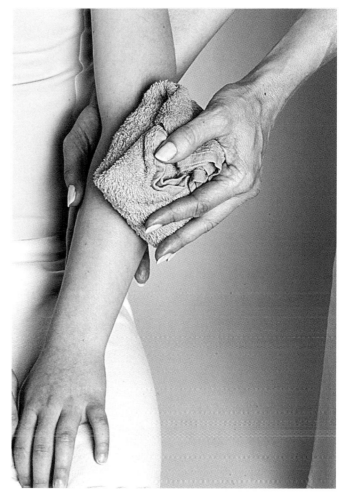

Hold a cold compress on the bite area.

 Seek urgent medical attention for spider bites that cause severe poisoning symptoms.

Scorpions

Scorpions lurk in cool, dark places. Children may be stung when playing near woodpiles or pulling bark off trees. Poisonous scorpions are recognizable by their small pincers and large tails. The venom is injected through a sting at the point of the tail. Most bites that appear 'out of nowhere' are caused by scorpions.

Signs of a scorpion sting

Although most stings cause only severe local pain, some may cause muscle pains, weakness, coma and convulsions.

✚ FIRST AID Apply ice or a cold compress to the sting. This will relieve pain and slow down the spread of venom. If the child does not develop any signs of systemic poisoning, wash the sting with soap and water, and watch for signs of infection. Seek urgent medical attention if the child develops a generalized rash or other symptoms after a scorpion bite. Most hospital emergency rooms carry a supply of anti-venom to neutralize the poison.

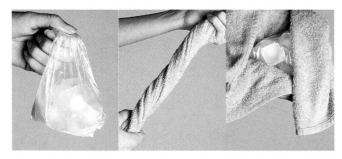

Wrap ice in a damp towel to make a cold compress.

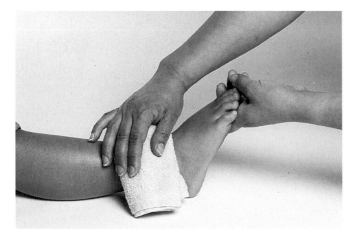

Apply the cold compress to a scorpion sting to relieve pain and inhibit the spread of the venom.

Ticks

These small brown insects are plentiful in wooded areas and farmland. They attach to the skin with hook-like mouthparts and suck blood. Most tick bites are harmless, but some (for example, the Australian scrub tick) contain venom that can cause a general paralysis which only clears up on removal of the tick. Other ticks contain bacteria and can transmit infections when they bite.

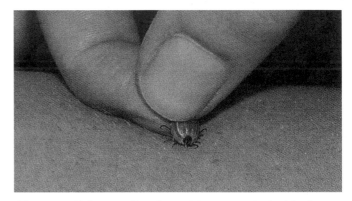

Remove ticks gently; do not leave parts behind.

Tick-bite fever

This is caused by the rickettsia micro-organism and is common in African countries. The bite is followed 10 to 14 days later by fever, a rash, headaches and painful swelling of lymph glands near the bite – usually the neck, armpit or groin. The area around the bite itself may become inflamed. A dark scab in the middle of the bite is characteristic of tick-bite fever.

Lyme disease

This infection is caused by bacteria carried and transmitted by the deer tick. Most infections occur in summer. Within days a red rash appears around the tick bite, with fever, headache, muscle and joint pains appearing weeks or even months later. If Lyme disease is not diagnosed and treated, the child may develop muscle paralysis and other severe complications.

FIRST AID Remove the tick by gripping it close to the skin, and pulling gently but firmly with your fingers or a pair of tweezers. Too much force can leave the mouth parts of the tick embedded, and this can result in a persistent sore. Carefully check the child's body for additional ticks.

Seek medical attention if:

- your child becomes unwell in any way in the weeks following a tick bite (both tick-bite fever and Lyme disease can be successfully treated with antibiotics).

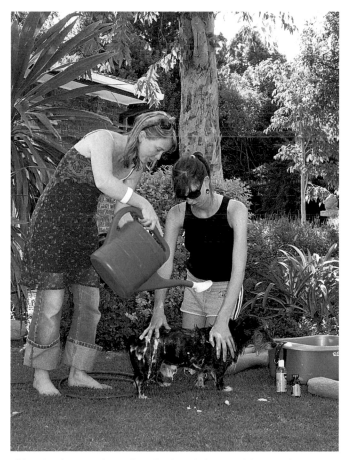

Check domestic animals for ticks and have them dipped or dosed regularly.

Fleas and bedbugs

Papular urticaria (*see* Urticaria, page 139) from insect bites is common in the hot months. Repeated bites from fleas or bedbugs may result in hypersensitivity and severe itching at the site of both fresh and old bites. The spots often become infected from scratching, frequently with streptococci.

FIRST AID Crotamiton™ cream applied three times daily to the itchy spots is soothing and antiseptic.

A blitz on fleas within the house is essential. Spray mattresses, skirting boards and cracks in the floor with insecticide. Keep your house as dust-free as possible. Ask your veterinary surgeon to dip your domestic animals or use an effective flea-killer, particularly during the warmer months of the year.

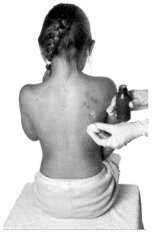

Calamine lotion helps to soothe itchy bites.

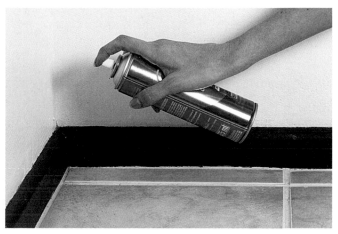

Spray skirting with insecticide to keep fleas at bay.

SNAKE BITES

Worldwide, there are nearly 3000 varieties of snake, but only about 300 are venomous, and even fewer are a danger to humans. Sea and land snakes are generally non-aggressive unless molested, and bites to children are uncommon. Adders and vipers (including the rattlesnake) may be trodden on accidentally and strike at the ankles and lower legs. The cobra rears up when cornered and will strike higher on the body; the spitting cobra is able to eject venom with force and accuracy at the eyes, causing severe pain and often permanent blindness.

Familiarize yourself with the types of snakes present in your area and find out whether anti-venom is available at your local hospital. (Species of dangerous snakes vary so much from region to region that this book cannot do justice to them. We advise the reader to obtain a good illustrated country-specific book on snakes and snake bite, as a companion to this book.)

Venomous snakes usually have fangs, large heads, and elliptical eyes.

There are three main types:
1. *Cytotoxic (adders and spitting cobras)* – these cause local tissue damage, resulting in large, painful or infected ulcers at the site of the bite.
2. *Neurotoxic (cobras, black and green mamba, rinkhals)* – these affect the nervous system, causing slurring of speech, drooling, muscle weakness and breathing difficulty.
3. *Haematoxic (boomslang, birdsnake)* – these cause generalized bleeding.

Non-venomous snakes usually have teeth instead of fangs, small heads and round eyes. Their bites can become infected, and some of these snakes even leave teeth behind in the wound. Others may leave tiny scratch marks or irregular lacerations on the skin, instead of the characteristic puncture marks of the venomous snakes.

Snake features

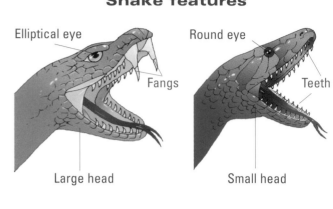

Poisonous snake

Non-poisonous snake

✚ FIRST AID

- A snake bite is extremely frightening, so calm and reassure the child.
- Keep her still – movement increases the spread of venom to other parts of the body.
- Remove any jewellery or tight clothing from the bitten area in case swelling develops.
- Apply a firm overlapping bandage to the limb, starting over the bite site, and winding it as far up the limb as possible to the armpit or groin. This will reduce the spread of venom through the lymphatic system.

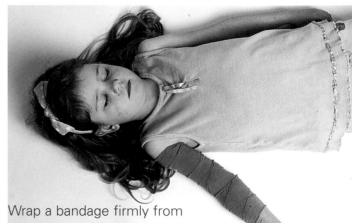

Wrap a bandage firmly from the bite up to the armpit.

- Do not clean the bite area. A venom sample may be taken to help identify which anti-venom should be used.
- Transport the child to hospital on a stretcher if possible to limit movement. Watch carefully for breathing difficulties on the way and commence basic life support if necessary.

Even a small amount of snake venom can be fatal in a child. so it is best to treat all snake bites as dangerous, and get the child to a hospital as soon as you have administered first aid.

MARINE CREATURES

Children can be stung by a variety of venomous fish, sea snakes and shellfish when exploring rock pools during beach vacations, or accompanying adults on fishing trips. Supervise children carefully during these outings, and teach them to inspect jellyfish, spiny fish, sea urchins and other sea creatures with their eyes only.

The large group of venomous sea creatures known as jellyfish includes the Portuguese man-of-war, bluebottle, sea anemone, sea nettle and sea louse, found in warm coastal waters around the world and often washed ashore. They appear dead when washed up by the tide, but the sting remains alive and is dangerous for some time.

All varieties possess tentacles that fire off toxin to paralyze their prey. The box jellyfish commonly found on the northeast coast of Australia has a toxic sting which is extremely dangerous. Emergency services at coastal resorts where this species is commonly found will usually have a specific antivenom for the box jellyfish.

Most popular beach resorts have signs that warn you about any dangerous marine life likely to be found in the area, so be observant.

Signs of jellyfish sting

- intense pain and burning at the sting site;
- a raised, red, whip-like swelling;
- an itchy rash that erupts one to two weeks after the sting;
- muscle pains, breathing difficulty and shock.

FIRST AID Call for help and begin basic life support (*see* pages 18–27) if the child has any breathing difficulty. Wash the sting area with vinegar for at least one minute. This inhibits the firing of toxin from any tentacles still adhering to the skin. Carefully remove these tentacles. Apply cold compresses to the skin for pain relief.

Seek immediate medical attention if the child shows any signs of generalized toxic effects. When calling the ambulance, mention that jellyfish anti-venom may be required.

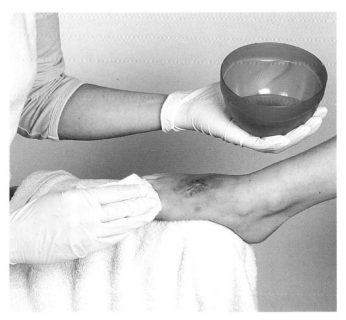

Wash a jellyfish sting with vinegar to restrict the poison from being fired from any leftover tentacles.

NEAR-DROWNING

Drowning is the second most common cause of injury-related death in children. Every child is vulnerable, but children under four years of age are especially so; they account for 80% of fatal drowning accidents.

PREVENTING DROWNING

A small child can drown in any liquid deep enough to cover the mouth and nose – as little as 2.5cm (1in) is a hazard. Bathtubs are the main water hazard to children under one year of age, while swimming pools and spas are a risk to toddlers and older children. In particular, any child with special needs or with a neurological disorder such as epilepsy should be introduced to water with the utmost care and always supervised one-on-one by an adult.

The most vital factor in preventing drowning in children is adult supervision – whether the child can swim or not. Many safety measures can substantially reduce the risk of accidental immersion in water but none can substitute for constant adult vigilance (*see* Water Safety, page 15).

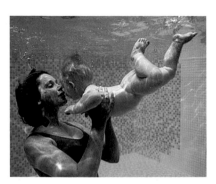

From five months of age, professional lessons can make less likely for your baby to drown.

How children drown
Within seconds

You may see a child drowning, but you will not hear him. This is because instead of kicking and screaming (as seen in the movies), he simply struggles to breathe.

Any water that passes through the mouth before the child sinks is more likely to enter the stomach than the lungs. As she sinks and water enters the throat, breathing stops, the windpipe is closed off, and the heart rate slows. These reactions are all part of a protective reflex called the diving reflex, which we share with other mammals.

Within two minutes

Lack of oxygen for two minutes or more will cause loss of consciousness. The child may start to breathe again, in which case water, and anything floating in the water, will enter the lungs. From this stage onward, the chance of survival rapidly deteriorates.

Breath holding, inhalation of water and suffocation all contribute to progressive oxygen starvation – the main cause of death from drowning.

Within four minutes

Lack of oxygen for four minutes or more will result in permanent brain damage. Tragically, this is the outcome for one child out of every five children who survive near-drowning.

Associated injuries

Hypothermia may complicate near-drowning in any child submerged in very cold water for even a short time (*see* Hypothermia, pages 80–81).

Head and neck injuries should always be suspected in a child who might have dived or fallen into shallow water (less than 3m, or 9ft), particularly if the child is unconscious when she is rescued (*see* Head and Neck Injuries, pages 53–56).

After rescue

Delayed complications may occur in children who are successfully rescued and resuscitated. These include lung infection, brain swelling and hypoglycaemia (a fall in the blood sugar level).

The effects and outcome of near-drowning are the same whether a child falls into salt water or fresh.

In cases of near-drowning, it is all about rescue, resuscitation and speed. If there is a single situation where the speed and skill with which you provide basic life support makes a difference, it is near-drowning. Rapid restoration of ABC can save a life that might otherwise be lost, and reduce the chance and degree of permanent brain damage in survivors.

Here is how you do it.

➕ **FIRST AID**   The S-A-F-E approach

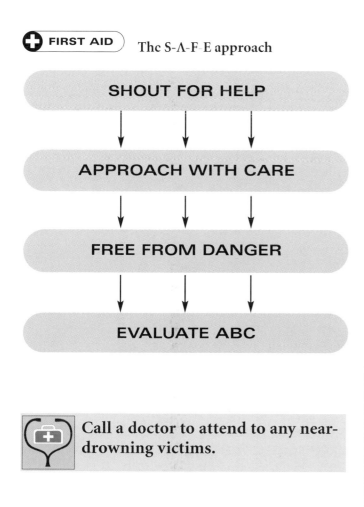

SHOUT FOR HELP

⬇   ⬇   ⬇

APPROACH WITH CARE

⬇   ⬇   ⬇

FREE FROM DANGER

⬇   ⬇   ⬇

EVALUATE ABC

Call a doctor to attend to any near-drowning victims.

Shout for help

If you cannot swim, call for someone else to rescue the child from deep water. Only experienced lifeguards or competition-fit swimmers should attempt to rescue anyone from the open sea.

Approach with care

Never put your own life at risk. If you cannot swim, find someone who can. If the child has fallen through cracking ice, do not do so yourself. You are no use to a drowning child if you are drowning yourself!

Free from danger

Get the child out of the water as quickly as possible to reduce the risk of hypothermia and exhaustion. If you rescue a child in water far from land, keep him face-up and begin rescue breathing while you swim for shore.

Older, conscious children may be pulled from frozen water, streams or pools using a rope, towel or anything long enough and easy to grip.

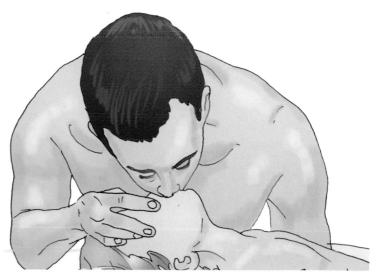

Get the child out of the water and begin rescue breathing (see page 24) as soon as possible.

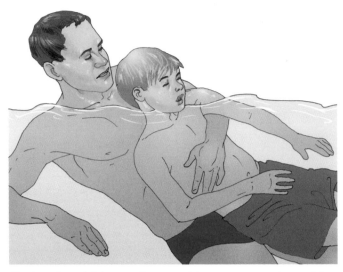

Swim the child to safety, making sure you keep his head above water.

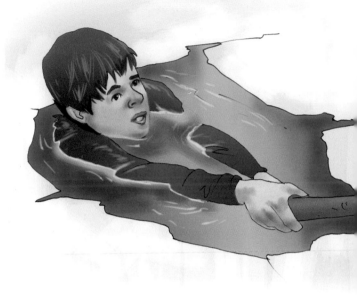

Evaluate the ABCs

Continue resuscitation until help arrives (*see* The ABC of Life Support, pages 18–27). Consider possible head or neck injury (*see* Head and Neck Injuries, pages 53–56) and avoid neck movement in an unconscious child.

Check for signs of hypothermia. Keep the child warm by removing wet clothing and wrapping her in a blanket or dry towels. Because of the risk of head or neck injury, as well as delayed complications, all near-drowning survivors should be examined by a doctor after being successfully resuscitated.

Do not give food or drink to a child who has been submerged in water. The stomach may be filled with air (because the child has been gasping) and swallowed water, so vomiting commonly occurs after rescue. If she is not fully conscious, vomited stomach contents may pass into the lungs, aggravating the injury and increasing the risk of pneumonia.

Do not try to pump water out of the lungs as often shown in the movies. The key to resuscitation is getting oxygen in – not water out.

But the most important thing of all is: do not let drowning happen in the first place!

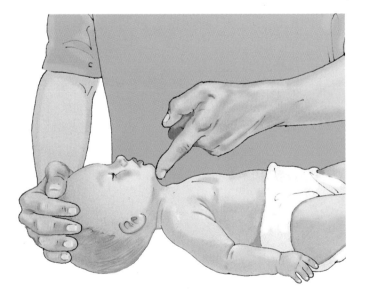

1. Open the airway using the chin lift.

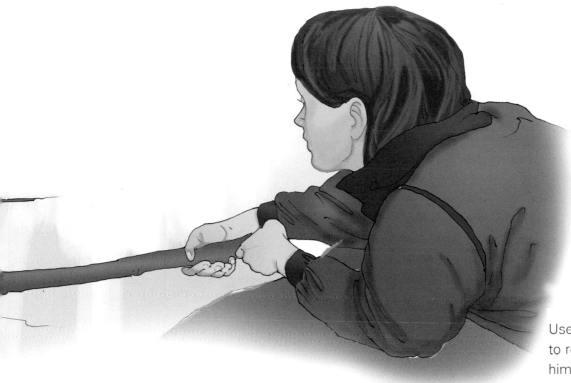

Use a stick, rope or towel to reach the child and pull him out of freezing water.

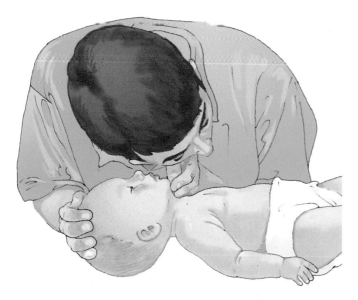

2. Look, listen and feel for breathing.

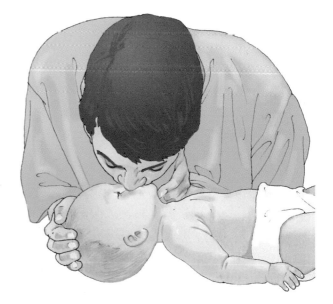

3. If he is not breathing, give up to five rescue breaths.

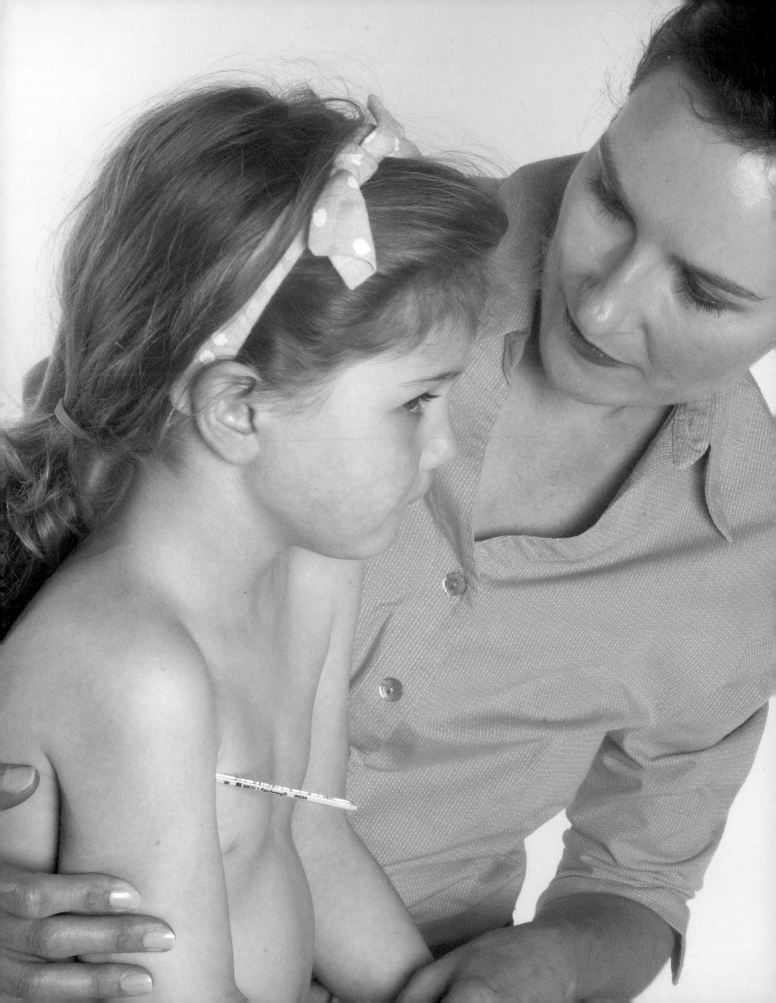

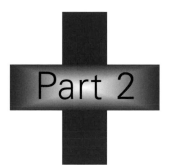

First Aid for
Medical Conditions

MEDICAL EMERGENCIES

- Is your baby experiencing any illness in the first four weeks of life? Illness in the first month could be serious.
- Does your child have a temperature over 40°C (104°F)?
- Is he refusing all feeds, including breast milk?
- Is he tired, listless and drowsy, refusing to play, not smiling, just staring ahead? Does he cry when touched or moved? Is he unable to sleep? Crying constantly? These symptoms may indicate severe pain or illness.
- Does he cry or push your hand away when you press gently on his tummy?
- Is his scrotum tender or swollen? This may indicate a twisted testis (*see* Torsion of the Testis, page 130).
- Does he have any difficulty breathing? Is there a crowing sound on breathing in?
  Is there wheezing?
  Is there rapid breathing? (*see* Breathing, page 19).
- Is there a drawing in of the lower chest?
- Is there a blue or grey colour to the lips?
- Is there inability to swallow, or drooling?
- Is he not walking when previously able to? Or limping?
- Is he dehydrated? (*see* Signs of Dehydration, page 122).
- Is the neck sore or stiff?
- Are there small blood spots or bruises in the skin? (*see* Rashes and Spots, pages 131–141).

SYMPTOMS REQUIRING IMMEDIATE MEDICAL HELP

As with minor injuries, illnesses are part of growing up. Colds, sore throats and diarrhoea are in a sense necessary because they help children develop immunity against infections. Nevertheless, the minor problems of infancy and early childhood can cause parents considerable anxiety. This section will help you understand and cope with common childhood illnesses – and to know when to get professional help.

Severe symptoms such as bleeding, unconsciousness or convulsions are obvious to anyone, but milder symptoms may not initially seem important. In the box on the left is a list of some that could mean your child is seriously ill or in pain and needs medical attention as soon as possible.

Pain and discomfort in children

If your child can talk to you and describe her feelings, it is easy to tell something is wrong, but if she is very young it is less easy. Consider five aspects of her behaviour to decide whether she is not her usual self:

- **Sleep pattern.** Is she sleeping well? Or is she waking at frequent intervals, or constantly awake?
- **Crying.** Does she moan or whimper, or cry steadily, or scream?
- **Activity.** Is she peaceful and contented? Or is she fussy and restless, or thrashing about? Or is she irritable or lethargic?
- **Feeding.** Is she feeding normally or regularly refusing feeds?
- **Can you distract her?** If she is crying or unhappy, can you distract or console her easily? If not, she may be ill or in pain and not just being 'difficult'.

FEVER

What is a fever?

A fever is a temperature above 38°C (100.4°F). The normal body temperature ranges between 36°C (96.8°F) and 37°C (98.6°F).

A raised temperature is a likely sign of illness, and the cause is generally an infection due to a virus or bacterium. Fever is one of the body's ways of attacking infection. It is in itself only an emergency if:

- there is fever in a baby under three months;
- the fever is excessively high – over 40°C (104°F);
- the fever causes a convulsion.

The most common cause of fever in children is an infection of the upper respiratory tract (colds, flu and tonsillitis). Fever and generally 'feeling rotten' are often the only initial symptoms – runny nose, sore throat, earache or cough may only develop after a day or two.

Some other possible causes are:

- pneumonia;
- a rash caused by a virus;
- mumps;
- a bowel infection;
- a urinary tract infection;
- heatstroke (see page 79).

Fever in an infant may indicate a germ in the blood stream (bacteraemia) or early meningitis.

✚ FIRST AID   To bring the child's temperature down you can give liquid paracetamol (acetaminophen) in the dosage recommended by a pharmacist. Do not give it more often than eight-hourly. Never give aspirin to children, except on a doctor's advice.

Remember fever is there for a purpose. It does not need to be brought down unless the child's temperature is very high – that is, above 39°C (102.2°F) – or if he is uncomfortable, or cannot sleep. Do not wake him to take his temperature or to dose him; sleep is a great healer!

Do not dress the child too warmly or cover him with too many blankets. Give him frequent drinks (for example, water or fruit juice) in small amounts. Finally, sponge him with lukewarm water if his temperature rises above 40°C (104°F).

 Get medical help if:

- the infant is younger than four months;
- there is rapid breathing (see Pneumonia, page 106);
- the child loses consciousness or has a convulsion;
- there is any rash;
- there is persistent vomiting or a stiff neck;
- the fever lasts for more than three days.

TAKING THE TEMPERATURE

Measure your child's temperature with a mercury or digital thermometer in the armpit. Do not place it under the tongue if the child is younger than seven. Alternatively, use a temperature strip on the forehead, but remember when you take a skin temperature to add 0.6°C (1°F) to get the true body temperature.

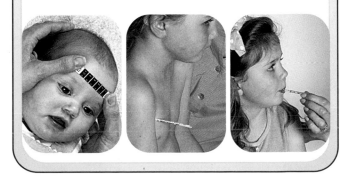

RESPIRATORY TRACT AND LUNG DISORDERS

The air we breathe passes through the nostrils, past the larynx, and down the trachea and bronchial tubes, which become progressively smaller until they reach the lungs. The most common causes of respiratory disorders are viral and bacterial infections that can affect any part of the respiratory tract. Young children are particularly prone to these infections as their immune systems are so immature. Allergic disorders such as asthma are also common in children.

COLDS AND FLU

All young children catch **colds** regularly, as often as five or six times a year. You will no doubt know the symptoms: a scratchy feeling in the throat, runny nose, sneezing, coughing and, in babies, a fever. A cold is particularly distressing for a baby, and the blocked nose makes it difficult for you to feed him. Colds are caused by viruses and usually clear up in three or four days.

Flu (or influenza) is an upper respiratory infection caused by the influenza virus. The symptoms are more severe than they are in the common cold – high fever, muscle aches, headache, tiredness and weakness – and they last longer.

Unfortunately, colds and flu are sometimes complicated by bacterial infection, which may lead to ear infection, sinusitis or pneumonia.

✚ FIRST AID for a cold

Where possible, keep infants out of close contact with anyone with a cold. Give more fluids than usual, in frequent small quantities. Paracetamol (acetaminophen) in liquid or tablet form will bring the temperature down and make the child feel better.

You can use a bulb aspirator to unblock your baby's nose. Saline nose drops are also helpful. Get a sterile saline (salt) solution from your pharmacist for this purpose.

The best decongestant is humidified air. Use a vaporizer, or place a wet towel near a heater. You can also boil a kettle in the room to create steam – but make sure it is safe! Alternatively, take the child to the bathroom and run the hot water tap. Stay with her to avoid accidental scalding.

A good home remedy is a teaspoon or two of honey or syrup and a little lemon juice in a cup of warm water, given three times a day. We do not recommend that you use nasal decongestants, whether in nose drop, spray or oral form. (They can have a rebound effect, making the problem worse.) Do not give the child cough suppressants. The cough helps get rid of mucus in the throat.

Colds generally clear up on their own and there is no need for antibiotics. However, see the doctor if there is prolonged fever or earache or if the symptoms do not clear up within a few days.

✚ FIRST AID for flu

Treat as for a cold, except in cases as listed on page 105.

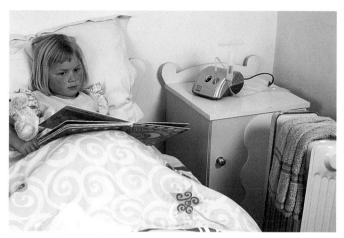

Use a vaporizer and a wet towel on a heater to humidify the air and ease breathing.

Seek medical attention if:

- the child's temperature is above 40°C (104°F);
- there is abnormally fast breathing (*see* Pneumonia, page 106);
- the child is drowsy or unwilling to feed.

Flu is dangerous in a child under two or with a chronic illness. After a dose of flu a child should not take part in vigorous games for two weeks.

For advice about flu vaccines, *see* Immunization, pages 142–144.

SINUSITIS

The sinuses are air spaces in the cheekbones and above and behind the nose, linked to the nasal passages. A cold may be followed by acute sinusitis, an infection that causes thick yellow nasal secretions, bad breath, a cough, fever, and pain and tenderness over the affected sinuses – usually the forehead or cheeks. A child may get sinusitis repeatedly over a long period, with recurrent fever and ill health. If untreated, infection can spread beyond the sinuses, causing serious complications.

 FIRST AID Decongestant (vasoconstrictor) nasal drops help to open up the narrow openings into the inflamed sinuses. Do not use them for more than three or four days; they may make the congestion worse when the effect of the drops wears off.

If your doctor prescribes an antibiotic, ensure the child completes the full course so that the infection does not recur.

If you suspect sinusitis, consult your doctor.

Diagram of the sinuses

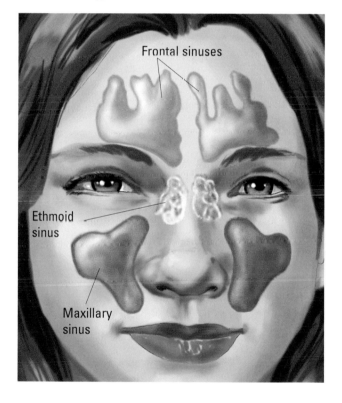

Frontal sinuses

Ethmoid sinus

Maxillary sinus

Make your own nose or eye drops by thoroughly dissolving half a teaspoon of clean salt in a cup of warm, previously boiled water.

PNEUMONIA

Pneumonia is an inflammation of one or both lungs due to bacteria, viruses or other organisms. It often develops after a cold, when germs in the nose and throat are carried into the lungs, or it may complicate another illness, such as whooping cough or measles.

In babies or infants it may also indicate an underlying problem in the lung, such as inhaled feed. In toddlers, it may be the first sign of obstruction by an inhaled foreign body (*see* Foreign Bodies, pages 68–70). Pneumonia is generally more severe in children who are malnourished or have a chronic illness.

Pneumonia may be complicated by painful inflammation of the membranes of the lung (pleurisy) or fluid collecting around the lung.

A child with pneumonia:

- is feverish and unwell;
- has a persistent, initially dry, cough;
- may cough up brownish or blood-stained sputum;
- breathes rapidly (*see* page 19 for a table of breathing rates in infants and children);
- may or may not have pain on breathing.

 Take the child to hospital if there is:

- indrawing of the chest on breathing;
- blueness of the lips and tongue;
- marked drowsiness;
- inability to feed;
- convulsions.

After consulting a doctor, treat the child at home unless she is very ill. Give her food frequently in small amounts, and paracetamol (acetaminophen) syrup in the recommended dosage to relieve fever and headache.

The doctor may prescribe an antibiotic. In an uncomplicated case the child should be better in a few days. A chest X-ray must be done after recovery to check there is no residual disease or underlying abnormality.

WHOOPING COUGH (PERTUSSIS)

Whooping cough is an acute and highly infectious disease caused by a bacterium, *Bordetella pertussis*. The illness is usually prolonged – it has been called the 90-day cough.

It starts as a mild cold with a cough, especially at night. These symptoms worsen, and at the end of the second week spasms of severe coughing develop, during which the child becomes red in the face and saliva drools from the mouth. Each spasm ends with a crowing indrawing of breath – the whoop – and there may be vomiting. In very young infants the breathing may stop altogether at the end of the spasm.

During the convalescent phase the whooping gradually disappears. It may return over a number of months, whenever the child develops a fresh cold. The spasms are exhausting for the child and can cause haemorrhages in the eyes and other complications, including pneumonia, marked weight loss from poor appetite and vomiting, and even (rarely) brain damage.

✚ FIRST AID If your child has been in contact with someone with whooping cough, or any prolonged cough, get medical help at the first sign of any illness. An antibiotic can stop whooping cough at this stage.

Once the whooping starts, only time will stop it. Get medical help as soon as possible.

Whooping cough is preventable. Make sure your baby is fully immunized at the correct times (*see* Immunization, pages 142–144). Immunization does not prevent all cases, but the illness is likely to be much less severe if it does occur.

BREATHING DIFFICULTIES

One of the most common breathing problems is the blocked nose associated with the common cold. This is very troublesome to infants, who cannot breathe through their mouths or blow their noses. Enlarged adenoids cause snoring at night and continuous mouth breathing, while croup is a difficulty with breathing in, resulting in a crowing sound and barking cough. Infection of the bronchial tubes causes wheezing, which is difficulty in breathing out. Lung infection shows itself by rapid and difficult breathing. Finally, complete obstruction to breathing results in asphyxiation – an extreme emergency.

ASPHYXIATION

Young infants are particularly vulnerable to asphyxiation – breathing being obstructed by food or a small object. Common offenders are such things as a peanut, a piece of sausage, or an uninflated balloon. A baby can also suffocate by getting a plastic bag over his nose and mouth, or his head stuck between the side of the cot and the mattress or between the cot slats. A baby who is choking will be red in the face, or blue, and he will be unable to cry because he is struggling to breathe.

(*See also* The Choking Child, pages 28–30, and Foreign Bodies, pages 68–70.)

Correct sleeping position for babies

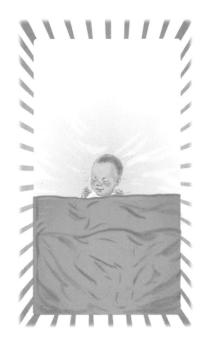

Put your baby to sleep on his back, with his feet near the bottom of the cot. This prevents him from slipping down under the blankets, where he may become overheated or even suffocate.

ANAPHYLACTIC SHOCK

This is a severe allergic reaction to a food, such as nuts or seafood, an insect sting, or a medication such as penicillin. Though uncommon in children, it is dangerous when it does occur.

The reaction comes on a few minutes after exposure. There is a sudden feeling of anxiety, followed by:
- a generalized itchy rash;
- burning of the lips and throat;
- swelling around the eyes;
- increasing difficulty with breathing;
- shock and collapse; and even
- loss of consciousness.

FIRST AID Sometimes shock and collapse come on very suddenly without any of the other warning signs. Get medical help immediately. Call for help or ask someone to summon an ambulance.

Place the child in a semi-sitting position to ease the breathing. If she loses consciousness begin basic life support (*see* The ABC of Life Support, pages 18–27).

A doctor or nurse can give her an injection of adrenalin, which is usually rapidly effective. Other drugs may also be given.

When your child is better, consult a paediatrician or allergy expert to try to find out what she is allergic to. If you know she is allergic to something she should wear a wrist band (MedicAlert) indicating this. Keep an adrenalin injection (Epipen™) at hand in case of emergency.

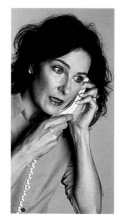

Call for medical help if the child collapses.

CROUP

Croup is an acute viral infection, most commonly affecting children aged six months to three years. It affects the upper airway, usually starting with cold symptoms and fever. This may be followed within a few days by inflammation of the upper windpipe just below the voice box, causing a hoarse barking cough and breathing difficulty. Typically, the child with croup makes a crowing sound, particularly on crying. In older children the croup virus simply causes hoarseness and cough (laryngitis).

Croup tends to come on at night and is always very frightening to both child and parents. The progress of this illness is unpredictable, and it is important to recognize the symptoms as soon as possible and take appropriate action.

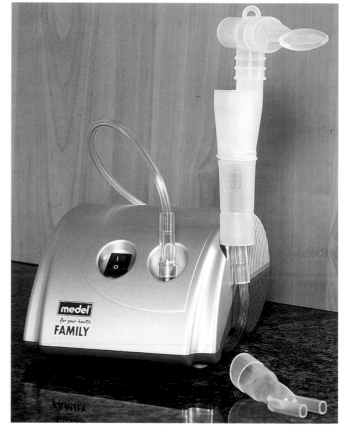

If your child has difficulty breathing, invest in a nebulizer to humidify the atmosphere.

 FIRST AID Be calm, and stay with the child – crying usually makes the symptoms worse. Give a dose of paracetamol (acetaminophen). Give him warm drinks, and humidify the air to ease breathing (*see* Respiratory Tract and Lung Disorders, pages 104–106).

Get medical help if:

- the child does not improve, or cannot feed normally;
- there is indrawing of the lower chest on breathing in;
- the lips, tongue or skin look blue;
- the child appears exhausted, or breathing suddenly becomes shallow.

Croup can be greatly eased by an aerosol or injection of adrenalin, or other medication which a doctor may decide to use.

A very dangerous form of croup, acute epiglottitis, is caused by a bacterium, *Haemophilus influenzae*. It should be suspected if:

- there is high fever;
- there is complete loss of voice;
- there is drooling and inability to swallow;
- the child is only comfortable in a sitting position.

Fortunately epiglottitis has become rare since the introduction of immunization to prevent it. If your child shows these symptoms, get him to a hospital or clinic at once.

BRONCHITIS

Bronchitis is an inflammation of the larger airways (bronchi). It may follow a cold. Thick secretions and spasm of these airways make the child cough and wheeze (have difficulty in breathing out). There may or may not be fever. If a child develops bronchitis after every cold, it may be the first sign of asthma.

✚ FIRST AID   Encourage the child to drink in order to help to prevent dehydration. Humidify the air to ease breathing (*see* Respiratory Tract and Lung Disorders, pages 104–106).

Place the child face down over your knees and gently tap the back of the chest on each side with a cupped hand for a few minutes to help bring up the mucus. Or tickle her to make her laugh – this usually causes coughing. If the secretions are yellow, your doctor may prescribe an antibiotic. Do not give cough suppressants. A bronchodilator such as salbutamol eases the spasm and releases mucus. It is available on prescription as syrup, tablets or aerosol. Ask your pharmacist for dosage instructions.

The bronchial system

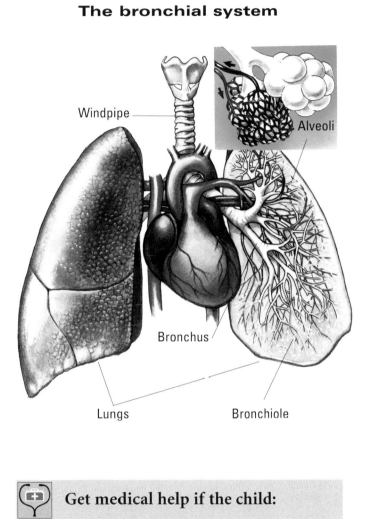

Windpipe

Alveoli

Bronchus

Lungs

Bronchiole

✚ Get medical help if the child:

- has difficulty breathing;
- is breathing rapidly (*see* Pneumonia, page 106);
- is exhausted.

BRONCHIOLITIS

This is an acute viral infection affecting the smallest airways (bronchioles) inside the lungs. It occurs mostly in infants under 12 months and can be a dangerous condition in very young or weak babies.

At the start the illness may resemble a cold. The baby then becomes increasingly distressed and feverish and may refuse feeds. There is a cough and breathing difficulty. The chest is bloated with air trapped in the lungs. The baby may stop breathing for a few seconds at a time.

Because the course of bronchiolitis is unpredictable, get medical help immediately if your child shows these symptoms. She may need oxygen therapy in hospital.

⊕ FIRST AID After the doctor has seen her, home treatment may include:

- giving plenty of fluids;
- humidifying the air to ease breathing (*see* Respiratory Tract and Lung Disorders, pages 104–106);
- giving paracetamol (acetaminophen) for the fever.

The child usually gets better within a week, but the cough can persist for much longer. There is no permanent damage to the lungs, but she may subsequently be prone to wheezing attacks.

See also Pneumonia and Whooping Cough, page 106.

ASTHMA

Asthma is a common condition affecting about one in 10 children, and is twice as common in boys. Only about half of the children who have asthma still have attacks after the age of 10 years.

The first symptom is usually a nagging cough, especially at night. Other symptoms are recurrent attacks of wheezing, tightness of the chest and shortness of breath, especially after exercise. Often the child has other allergies, such as hay fever or eczema, and other family members may be similarly affected.

Asthma is caused by a narrowing of the lung airways and accumulation of secretions. In a susceptible child, it may be brought on by excitement, infection, exercising in cold air, and allergy to house dust, pollens, pets, pollutants such as tobacco smoke, and some foods.

⊕ FIRST AID If your child has repeated attacks of coughing or wheezing, ask your doctor for a full assessment. She will rule out other causes of cough and wheezing, as well as doing tests for asthma.

Various medications are available for a child with asthma. You can teach him how to use them in an attack. You will need to assist a younger child. Relieving medicines are now usually given in the form of an inhaled spray or an aerosol, or nebulizer. Preventive medicines are also available. When given every day, they will prevent most attacks.

Keep your asthmatic child well away from tobacco smoke and any other kind of smoke.

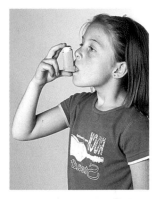

Asthma pumps must be kept handy.

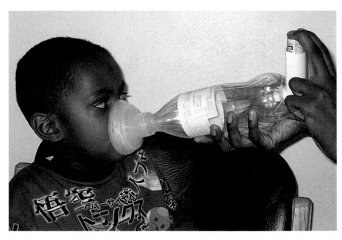

For young children use a spacer attached to the pump as they cannot synchronize breath intake with the puffs from the pump. A small plastic bottle makes an inexpensive spacer. Cut a hole in the bottom for the pump nozzle. The aerosol is pumped into the bottle at one end while the child breathes in at the other.

MOUTH, THROAT, NOSE AND EAR PROBLEMS

The nose and mouth are entry points for micro-organisms in the air we breathe and the fluids and food we ingest so, not surprisingly, nose and throat infections are the most common in children. The middle ear is an air-filled space closed to the outside by the eardrum. Its only exit is a narrow tube leading to the back of the nose. This tube is readily blocked by enlarged adenoids, when the child has a cold, or by abrupt changes in pressure caused by air travel – with resulting infection.

THRUSH

Thrush (*oral candida* or *monilia*) is a common fungal infection of the mouth in infants. You will see white patches on the tongue, inside the cheeks and sometimes in the throat. If severe, the condition causes some discomfort, and feeding may be affected. It can also cause severe nappy rash (*see* Nappy Rash, page 136). In older children thrush may develop after the administration of antibiotics, or the use of a nebulizer for asthma.

FIRST AID   Thrush can be cured with oral anti-fungal drops such as nystatin or by putting one drop of 1% acqueous gentian violet inside each cheek three times a day. If thrush is persistent, seek medical advice as it may be an early sign of immune deficiency.

MOUTH ULCERS AND COLD SORES

The herpes simplex virus that causes these is widespread in the community. In fact, most of us carry it unnoticed. Children infected with it for the first time may develop a very sore mouth and throat. The child is feverish, the throat is inflamed and there are many ulcers (blisters that have burst) inside the mouth. The gums are usually inflamed and swollen. Sometimes there are also cold sores (fever blisters) on the lips or around the mouth, and even on one or two fingers the child has sucked. This is a significant illness in children under five. They take seven to 10 days to get better and during this time feeding is very painful.

FIRST AID   In mild cases, control discomfort with tannic acid and lignocaine gel, or Dequadin Mouth Paint™ applied to the mouth ulcers; give paracetamol (acetaminophen) for the fever eight-hourly; give milk and bland fluids (preferably chilled) in small amounts at regular intervals, but not acidic fruit juices; give 5ml (one teaspoon) of a multi-vitamin mixture daily.

 For severe cases consult a doctor.

Some children get mouth ulcers from time to time without other symptoms. The cause is unknown. Rinsing the mouth with a mild salt solution may be soothing, or ask a pharmacist for a suitable medication.

Some also get recurrent cold sores on the lips – usually a minor complaint requiring no treatment. When they cause burning, discomfort or embarrassment, a doctor may prescribe a cream containing the anti-viral agent acyclovir to clear them more quickly.

HAND, FOOT AND MOUTH DISEASE

Other viruses can also cause sores in the mouth and throat. Hand, foot and mouth disease is a common viral infection that tends to occur in summer. It is generally a mild illness, starting with slight fever and a few ulcers in the mouth. After a day or two blisters appear on the hands and feet, and often on the knees. The blisters on the arms and legs usually disappear after three or four days.

⊕ FIRST AID   For treatment of mouth ulcers, *see* Mouth Ulcers and Cold Sores, page 111. Apply calamine lotion to blisters on hands and feet to relieve itching and dry out the sores.

MUMPS

Mumps is a common viral infection of the salivary glands, which lie in front of and below the ears, under the jaw and under the tongue. It starts with a day or two of fever, which may be so mild as to pass unnoticed in young children. The face becomes tender and swollen on one side or both, and there may be vomiting and headache. The swellings last for up to a week, after which the child rapidly gets better.

Feeding may be painful, especially anything acidic, so give him milk and bland foods.

⊕ FIRST AID   Mumps can be prevented by the MMR vaccine, so have your baby vaccinated (*see* Immunization, pages 142–144). Although it is generally a mild disease, consult a doctor.

Get medical attention urgently if the child has severe headache and vomiting, or abdominal or testicular pain. These symptoms may indicate a complication of the mumps virus.

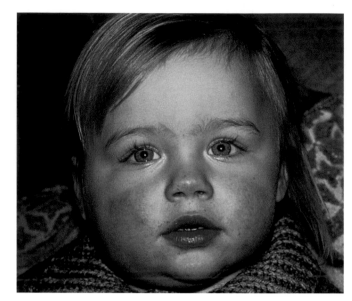

Swollen glands are characteristic of mumps.

TEETHING AND TOOTHACHE
Teething

This is a natural process and you should not attribute such symptoms as fever and diarrhoea to this cause. The appearance of the larger teeth (canines and molars) may be associated with some redness of the gums, discomfort and dribbling. Paracetamol (acetaminophen) syrup will relieve discomfort. Biting on a teething ring or a rusk may also help.

Toothache

Usually there are no symptoms until there is advanced tooth decay. Then there may be sensitivity to heat or cold and sometimes severe pain. Paracetamol (acetaminophen) syrup will help relieve the discomfort until you can see the dentist.

How to prevent tooth decay

- Encourage your child to brush twice a day with a fluoride toothpaste.
- Keep her diet low in sugar and do not allow sugary snacks between meals or last thing at night.

- Take her to the dentist for regular check-ups from age two and a half.
- If the water in your area is adequately fluorinated, no additional fluorine is needed. Ask your dentist about this.

(*See also* Tooth Injuries, pages 61–62.)

THROAT INFECTIONS
Pharyngitis and tonsillitis

The tonsils are situated on either side of the back of the throat. They serve two important functions: preventing harmful germs in the mouth and throat from entering the body, and making antibodies to fight infection. The adenoids, situated higher up in the back of the throat, do the same job.

In any throat infection in a child, whether due to viruses or bacteria, the tonsils will be enlarged and painful (tonsillitis), and the rest of the throat will usually be inflamed also (pharyngitis). A child with a very sore and red throat, high fever and enlarged tender glands at the angle of the jaw may have a bacterial infection ('strep throat', from streptococci), which requires antibiotics. But it is often impossible to tell a streptococcal throat infection from one caused by a virus, unless the doctor does a throat culture (to grow the germs so as to identify them). Consult a doctor, who will decide whether to prescribe an antibiotic.

As a general rule, you can make the child more comfortable with:

- paracetamol (acetaminophen) syrup, given four times a day;
- throat lozenges;
- gargling with salt water;
- cool liquids, such as fruit juice or milk, or ice cream, to relieve pain on swallowing.

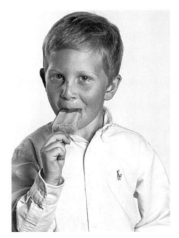

Sucking an ice lolly relieves a tender throat.

The tonsils

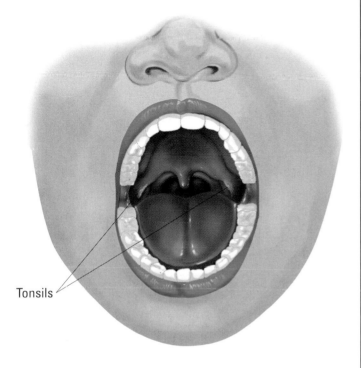

Tonsils

EARACHE

Earache commonly occurs in children between the ages of six months and two years. It is most often caused by an infection behind the eardrum and usually follows a cold, when the drainage tube from the middle ear to the back of the nose gets blocked. The fluid behind the drum raises the pressure and causes pain – and sometimes rupture – of the paper-thin eardrum. If this happens, the fluid or pus drains out, and pain is relieved. With proper treatment the eardrum reseals itself and full recovery should occur.

⊕ FIRST AID If you suspect earache consult a doctor. (Babies with ear infection may simply be irritable and sleepless, or frequently touch or rub the ear.)

Give prescribed medication exactly as directed and complete the full course. Give paracetamol (acetaminophen) for pain or if the fever is over 39°C (102.2°F). Do not put drops in the ear. (They obscure the eardrum and make it harder for the doctor to assess the infection.) Visit your doctor after two weeks to ensure the infection has cleared up and hearing is normal.

A child's middle ear cavities can become filled with thick, glue-like fluid, causing hearing loss. Drainage of the fluid may be required. A drainage tube (grommet) will be inserted through a small incision in the ear drum to allow fluid to escape and to equalize pressures in the middle ear. However, your doctor may want to wait three months as there is often spontaneous improvement.

NOSEBLEEDS

Nosebleeds are common throughout childhood. They are usually caused by picking the nose during colds, or vigorous sniffing or nose-blowing, and are frequent in children with hay fever (allergic rhinitis).

⊕ FIRST AID Get the child to sit, leaning forward, so that the blood can be spat out rather than swallowed. Have a basin handy for this. Swallowed blood is irritating to the stomach, so it is often vomited

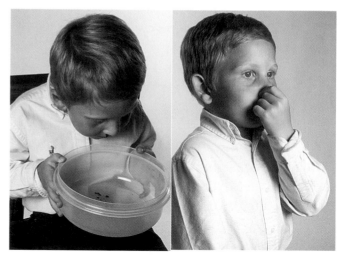

Lean forward over a bowl to spit out any blood. Pinch the nose shut and breathe through the mouth.

up. Let him blow his nose free of large clots. Then apply firm pressure by pinching the soft part of the nose against the central wall with your fingers, and maintain this pressure continuously for 10 minutes. Do not worry – he will breathe through his mouth. If bleeding continues, insert a piece of gauze soaked in vasoconstrictor nose drops (for example, phenylephrine) or coated with petroleum jelly, and continue pressure for a further 10 minutes. Leave the gauze in for a further 10 minutes before removing it.

A cold object placed on the back of the neck or elsewhere does not help to stop a nosebleed!

🩺 Get a medical opinion if:

- bleeding continues;
- the child feels dizzy or faints;
- there are any signs of bleeding elsewhere, such as bleeding spots in the skin;
- he has recurrent nose bleeds – repeated bleeding from one side may mean that a small vein needs to be cauterized.

EYE INFECTIONS

Common eye infections in children are conjunctivitis (affecting the mucous lining of the eyelids and eye), styes and blepharitis (affecting the eyelids). Fortunately, involvement of the eye itself, which is much more serious, is also much rarer. Get a medical opinion immediately if there is pain in the eye, marked sensitivity to light, and/or haziness of vision. There may be a scratch or sore on the cornea (the transparent part of the eye), a foreign body in the sclera (the white of the eye), or a problem within the eye itself. (*See also* Eye Injuries, pages 57–59.)

CONJUNCTIVITIS

Conjunctivitis (also called 'pink eye') is an infection of the thin membrane that covers the whites of the eyes and the inside of the eyelids. It may be caused by a virus, bacterium or, in the newborn, by a microorganism called chlamydia.

Viral conjunctivitis results in red eyes, irritation and watery discharge. In bacterial conjunctivitis, on the other hand, the discharge is yellow and the eyelashes are matted together after sleeping. Both eyes are almost always affected.

Other causes of red inflamed eyes include allergy – in which case the eyes are usually itchy as well – and irritation resulting from smoke or chlorine in swimming pools.

Conjunctivitis

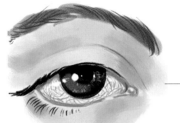

Viral conjunctivitis is also known as 'pink eye'

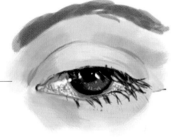

Bacterial conjunctivitis causes gummy sticky eyelashes

 FIRST AID   If the eyes are simply red without yellow discharge, bathe them frequently with mild salt solution (*see* box on page 105). Pour a few drops into each eye, wiping the excess away with cotton wool. Do this at least every hour while the child is awake. The conjunctivitis should clear in four to seven days.

If there is a sticky discharge, it is bacterial conjunctivitis, requiring antibiotic drops or ointment. Follow instructions from your doctor or pharmacist.

Always seek medical advice if:

- your baby (under six weeks) has inflamed eyes;
- only one eye is involved – this may mean the cornea has been scratched, or there is a foreign body in the eye (*see* Foreign Bodies in the Eye, pages 57–59);
- the eyelids become swollen;
- the child's vision is blurred.

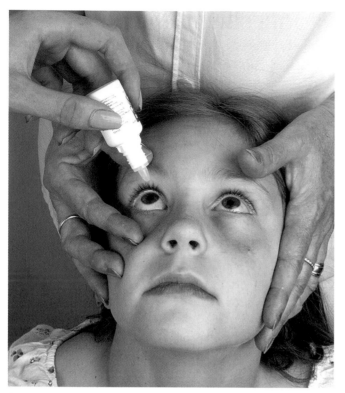

Putting eye drops into a young child's eyes may require two adults. One of you holds the child while the other puts them in.

APPLICATION TIPS

- If you cannot open the eyelids sufficiently, put drops in the inner corner of the eye with the child lying down and they will run into the eye itself.
- Put in drops every two hours.
- If you have difficulty applying ointment, apply it to the eyelid corners; it will reach the conjunctiva as it melts.
- Ointment is longer acting than drops; apply every four to six hours.

STYES

Styes are boils affecting the eyelashes. A stye will get better by itself, but you can help bring it to a head by applying heat.

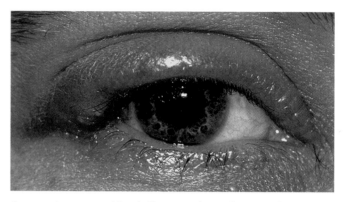

A stye is caused by inflammation of a hair follicle.

✚ FIRST AID

Warm a teaspoon in warm water (not too hot!) and get the child to apply it to her eye. Repeat this frequently. Applying an antibiotic eye ointment three times a day for a few days is a good idea. Get this from your pharmacist or doctor.

BLOCKED TEAR DUCTS

In infants and young children, the tube carrying tears from the eyes into the nose may be blocked on one or both sides, resulting in constant watering of the eye. There may be a bead of pus at the corner of the eye – sometimes mistaken for conjunctivitis.

✚ FIRST AID

Open a blocked duct by rolling your finger in the angle between nose and cheek bone, just below the eye. Though the problem usually resolves itself with time, see a specialist if it has not by the age of one year. Probing of the duct may be required.

HEADACHES

Headache is as common in children as in adults. It accompanies many childhood infections and is seldom the most troublesome symptom. But headache may also be the only, or earliest, indication of serious illness such as meningitis or other conditions that raise the pressure inside the head.

RECURRENT HEADACHES

Many children have recurring headaches with no apparent physical cause. Chronic non progressive headaches occur at irregular intervals, become more severe during the day and are brought on by stress or tiredness. Eye strain is often blamed, and it is a good idea to have your child's eyes tested. Sinusitis or a tooth infection may also be responsible.

Migraine headaches occur at regular intervals and there is often a history of migraine in the family. In a young child the main symptoms may be vomiting and/or abdominal pain. The classic visual effects that can precede a migraine – wavy patterns or dots to one side of the line of vision – occur only in older children.

If your child regularly gets headaches, first look for possible stresses within the family, school or peer group and deal with them. Then get a full medical assessment. Once the more serious causes are excluded (which is most likely) your doctor may diagnose migraine. Effective treatment is available to stop, even prevent, these headaches.

PROGRESSIVE HEADACHES

Headaches that steadily increase in severity are a different matter. These may be caused by raised pressure in the head, or high blood pressure. They are the only headaches that will wake a child from sleep. Effortless vomiting without preceding nausea is a particular danger sign. Get medical advice urgently.

MENINGITIS

Meningitis is an infection of the membranes around the brain, and may be caused by a variety of micro-organisms. The symptoms of viral and bacterial meningitis are similar in the early stages, but bacterial meningitis tends to be much more severe. In infants the symptoms may be vague – crying, restlessness, refusing feeds, vomiting, fever, or abnormal drowsiness, and sometimes convulsions. Older children can tell you they have a severe headache, cannot stand bright light or loud noises and have a painful stiff neck.

In one common and dangerous form (meningococcal meningitis) there may be bleeding spots in the skin – tiny red spots that do not blanch on pressure, or larger bruises (*see* Meningococcal Infection, page 135).

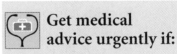 **Get medical advice urgently if:**

- a child complains of severe headache;
- she vomits persistently;
- she has a stiff neck;
- she is drowsy or lethargic;
- she has a convulsion;
- she has small bleeding spots in the skin.

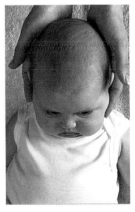

Tilting the head forward onto the chest will be painful if the child has meningitis.

CONVULSIONS AND SEIZURES

Convulsions and seizures are brief passing attacks of disturbed consciousness, sometimes accompanied by abnormal movements of limbs or body. There are many causes – sudden rise of temperature, low blood sugar or poisoning – so always consult your doctor if your child experiences a 'funny turn'.

FEBRILE CONVULSIONS

A convulsion (or fit) happens because of an abnormal electrical discharge in the brain, most commonly caused by a sudden rise in temperature brought on by an infection (a febrile convulsion).

These attacks are most frequent between the ages of six months and four years, when the brain is especially sensitive to rises in temperature. They are generally quite harmless, though frightening to parents and onlookers. The child will suddenly pass out, stiffen or develop twitching of the limbs, and the eyes will squint or roll upwards. She may feel hot, but sometimes the temperature rises so quickly you cannot immediately feel it in the skin. Most attacks last only a few minutes.

STAY CALM AND ASK FOR HELP

- Make sure the child's airway is clear and that she cannot injure herself against hard objects.
- Do not shake or slap her.
- Do not put anything in her mouth to prevent her biting her tongue.
- Take off her clothes and sponge her all over with lukewarm water, starting at the head.
- If her temperature is very high – above 40°C (104°F) – apply an ice pack or cool her with a fan.
- When the attack is over, put her in the recovery position (*see* page 23), with a light covering.

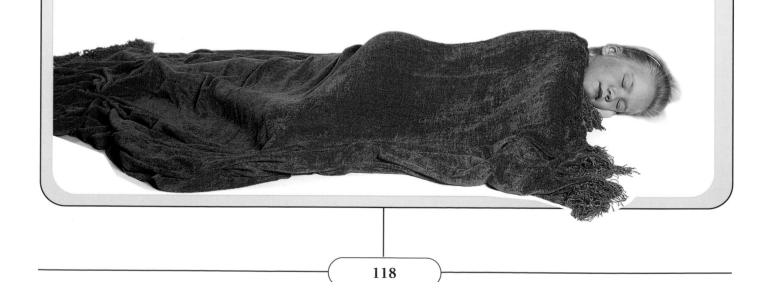

FIRST AID In most children this is a one-off event, but some may experience further convulsions with fever. In these cases, prevent attacks by giving a sedative (diazepam) rectally at the first sign of fever. Febrile convulsions generally have no ill-effects, and few children who have them later develop epilepsy.

> **Call the doctor if an attack lasts more than 10–15 minutes. Medication is needed.**

EPILEPSY

Epilepsy is a tendency (sometimes inherited) to have recurrent convulsions. It takes many forms and the diagnosis is not often made before the age of five. You should always get a specialist opinion to establish the cause and nature of recurrent fits. There are a number of effective medications to prevent convulsions or lessen their frequency and severity. An epileptic attack usually lasts only a few minutes.

 FIRST AID Follow the instructions for convulsions above. Do not try to stop the convulsion. Once it begins it cannot be stopped. If it lasts longer than a few minutes, or if the child is blue in the face or choking, get medical help immediately

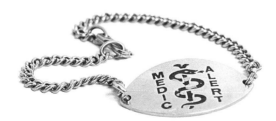

Every child with epilepsy should wear a MedicAlert wristband indicating the nature of the problem.

BREATH-HOLDING SEIZURES

When some young children start to cry, they hold their breath on breathing out and cannot breathe in. Their faces become red or purple and they may pass out for a few seconds. They then relax and normal breathing is restored. Loss of consciousness is due to slowing of the heart, in other words, to a temporary shortage of oxygen in the brain and not to an electrical discharge as in a convulsion.

These attacks are harmless and not related to epilepsy. They disappear as the child matures, usually by four years. Never allow fear of an attack to interfere with normal discipline. Ignore the attack, not the child!

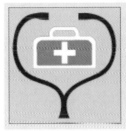 > **If you are concerned, call the doctor. She may want to check the child's blood count, as the attacks may be worsened by anaemia.**

FAINTING

This is sudden loss of consciousness with extreme pallor of the face, brought on by such things as an empty tummy combined with a stuffy room, standing in the heat, or a sudden fright. It is caused by a brief shortage of oxygen in the brain when the heart slows down or there is a drop in blood pressure. A child who faints regularly must be investigated by an expert.

STOMACH AILMENTS AND ABDOMINAL PAIN

Digestive system problems are frequent in children, second only to colds and sore throats. Although the common symptoms of vomiting and diarrhoea are upsetting, they are rarely persistent enough to be a serious threat to health. Other digestive disorders are less common but may cause chronic illness that can affect growth if left untreated.

VOMITING IN INFANTS

Vomiting is the forceful ejection of stomach contents. It should not be confused with regurgitation (posseting), which is an effortless spitting up after feeds, often with a wind. This is a normal feature in babies. The infant who possets and is otherwise well and gaining weight requires no special treatment.

 Consult a doctor if:

- regurgitation is frequent and copious;
- there is no gain in weight;
- there are any other symptoms, such as excessive crying or a cough.

A single vomiting episode is seldom cause for concern, but there are many possible reasons for vomiting in infants – if your baby keeps doing it you would be well advised to check with the doctor.

 FIRST AID   After a single episode of vomiting, give no feeds for one hour, then offer sips of clear fluids (such as water or fruit juice) every 15 minutes for one hour. Do not give any medications to stop the vomiting. Once there is no further vomiting, begin to introduce regular feeds in half quantities, then work up to the usual quantity.

 Get medical advice if:

- your baby has a fever above 38°C (100.4°F);
- he has a cough or diarrhoea;
- he vomits persistently;
- he is drowsy;
- your baby is dehydrated (*see* Signs of Dehydration, page 122);
- there is pain or the baby's abdomen is tender when you press it.

 Get urgent help if:

- the vomit is greenish or blood-stained;
- the vomiting is forceful and happens after every feed.

VOMITING IN CHILDREN

Some children are more prone to vomiting than others. Common, harmless causes of a single bout of vomiting are overeating, overexcitement or travel sickness.

In other cases vomiting may be the first sign of an infection. The commonest is a bowel infection (gastroenteritis), when vomiting is soon followed by the passing of loose, frequent stools. Sometimes contaminated food can cause an outbreak of vomiting in a number of people at the same time (known as food poisoning).

Other possible causes of vomiting

- ingestion of a toxic substance (*see* Poisoning, pages 85–88);
- acute appendicitis;
- an obstruction of the bowel;
- an infection of any kind (*see* in particular Meningitis, page 117);
- injury.

 FIRST AID Reassure the child and let her rest quietly. Do not give her any food or drink for an hour, and then offer her sips of water – or any non-fizzy clear drink – every 15 minutes. Never give any medications to stop vomiting. If there is no further vomiting, increase fluids steadily, and introduce solid food after six hours.

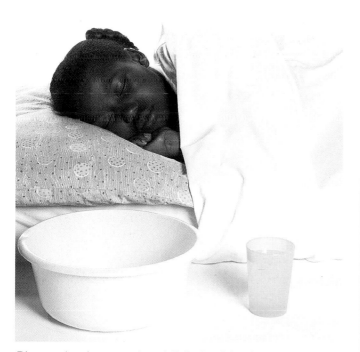

Place a basin near the child's bed for her to vomit into. Keep fluids nearby to prevent dehydration.

Take the child to the hospital if:

- she vomits persistently or for more than three hours;
- you suspect a head injury;
- she shows any symptoms of meningitis (*see* Meningitis, page 117);
- you suspect she has ingested a drug or poison;
- the urine is dark in colour;
- the vomit is greenish or blood-stained;
- there is any abdominal pain or tenderness (*see also* Hernia, page 124).

DIARRHOEA

Diarrhoea – abnormally frequent or liquid bowel movements – is a common symptom in children, most often due to gastroenteritis, an infection of the bowel caused by viruses or other organisms. The first signs may be tummy rumbling and vomiting and there may be cramping abdominal pain and tenderness. Gastro-enteritis caused by bacteria is more severe, and the stools may contain blood and mucus. When blood is present the term dysentery is used.

Diarrhoea may also be caused by infection elsewhere in the body, drugs or poisons accidentally swallowed, anxiety, or many other causes. The main danger is that if diarrhoea is severe, your child can become dehydrated.

FIRST AID Simply replace the fluid lost from the body. Do not use medications to make the stools firmer or less frequent – the body will take care of this in its own time.

If the diarrhoea is mild, the child can continue taking the usual feeds. Replace lost fluid by giving additional water, sugar and salts (*see* box on page 122). A toddler or young child who is still breast-fed can continue nursing. Continue normal feeds in frequent small amounts and give extra fluids.

For a child under two years give 50ml to100ml (a quarter to half a cup) of liquid after each loose stool. For an older child give 100ml to 200 ml (half to one cup) after each loose stool. If the child vomits, wait 10 minutes, then give the solution more slowly (for example, a teaspoonful every two to three minutes). If the child is very thirsty, give more fluid.

Do not give any medication to stop vomiting. Check the child's weight after recovery, and give her an extra feed a day for at least a week after she has recovered.

What fluids to give

Oral rehydrating solution (ORS) can be bought ready-mixed in a packet or as a prepared drink (Pedialyte™ or Resol™). These contain just the right amounts of salts and sugar and are the best way to replace fluid.

REHYDRATING SOLUTION

If you do not have an oral rehydrating solution, make your own sugar and salt solution by mixing eight level teaspoonsful of sugar and half a teaspoonful of table salt in one litre (two pints) of water (preferably boiled first and allowed to cool). A child older than two can be given non-fizzy fruit drinks instead, or add a little fruit juice to the salt solution for flavour.

Get medical help if:

- the diarrhoea lasts for five days or longer;
- the child is feverish;
- vomiting is continuous;
- the child is unable to drink;
- the child is lethargic or becomes drowsy;
- there is blood in the stools;
- breathing is rapid and deep;
- signs of dehydration increase (*see* below).

Recognizing severe diarrhoea
Signs of dehydration

You can recognize dehydration by the following signs:

- a dry mouth and tongue;
- sunken eyes;
- absence of tears when crying;
- decreased urination;
- lethargy and drowsiness;
- skin that goes back slowly when pinched.

DEHYDRATION CHECK

The pinch test is a very simple way to check for dehydration. Gently pinch the skin on the side of the abdomen and then let go. If the child is not dehydrated the skin will flatten immediately. If there is some dehydration, the fold will take a second or two to disappear. In cases of severe dehydration the fold of skin will stay raised for several seconds.

In the absence of these symptoms, a few days of diarrhoea are generally not cause for concern. But diarrhoea caused by a virus or bacterial infection may be contagious, so wash your hands well to avoid spreading germs, especially to those particularly at risk, such as other young children, the elderly, or people with weakened immune systems.

Preventing diarrhoea

Make sure you wash your hands well, particularly after nappy changes, before and after handling food (especially poultry) and after touching pets and cleaning aquariums or cat litter trays. Lessen the risk of food poisoning by thoroughly washing all kitchen and eating utensils, cleaning surfaces where you prepare or cook food, and cooking meat until it is cooked through and no longer pink.

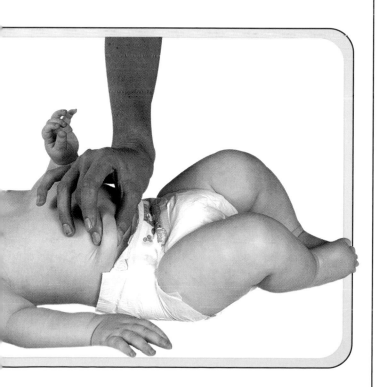

PAIN IN THE ABDOMEN

Occasional abdominal pains are common in children, but although there are some serious causes – and the pain is a symptom you should not disregard – most are minor upsets.

Abdominal pain in infants
Infantile colic

Colic in the first three months of life is probably just an extreme variety of the behaviour normal for this age, but can cause distress. It is characterized by regular vigorous crying, usually in the late afternoon or early evening. During these spells the infant cries, cannot be soothed, and draws up her legs or arches backward as though in pain. In all other respects she is well: she is not vomiting, she is gaining weight, and bowels, feeding and weight gain are normal. These spells have no lasting effect on the baby's health.

If the baby has a fever, or any symptoms other than the crying, the diagnosis is not infantile colic. If you are worried, consult a doctor or nurse.

✚ FIRST AID Ensure you are using the right techniques for feeding the baby and bringing up wind (burping). Avoid overfeeding; do not feed her every time she cries.

Allow her to suck a pacifier (dummy) – but remember to keep it clean – or, better still, to suck her fingers or thumb. This is a harmless practice. Carry her in a harness or sling at your front or back.

Do not stop breast feeding or change the feed formula. Milk allergy is seldom the cause of colic in infants under three months.

Do not use medications or sedatives.

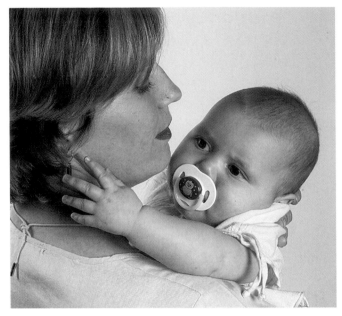

Sucking a pacifier helps to ease colic.

Hernia

A hernia, or rupture, is a weak spot in the abdominal wall that allows a segment of bowel to come through. The usual place for a hernia is the groin, in both boys and girls. The bowel can normally be pushed back with gentle pressure, but if it twists, or strangulates, it causes serious intestinal obstruction.

When a hernia strangulates, the baby shows sudden great discomfort:

- he refuses feeds;
- he vomits, and often the vomit is green in colour;
- the abdomen may become distended;
- there may be a firm tender lump in the groin, which cannot be pushed back with gentle pressure.

If your baby shows any of these symptoms, call an ambulance immediately.

The bulging of the navel (an umbilical hernia) is quite common in infants and usually disappears with time. These hernias very seldom strangulate. See a doctor if you are concerned.

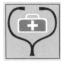 **These three conditions require urgent medical attention:**

1. Intestinal obstruction

Babies may develop a bowel obstruction because of some defect they were born with. Symptoms will be:

- sudden abdominal discomfort;
- refusing feeds;
- vomiting;
- abdominal distension.

2. Appendicitis

Very rarely a baby may develop appendicitis, and the symptoms may not be as apparent as in older children. You should suspect this if the baby has a fever and the stomach is swollen and tender.

3. Torsion of the testis

This can be the cause of abdominal pain in young male infants (*see* Torsion of the Testis, page 130).

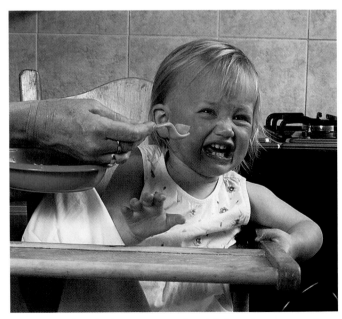

Refusing feeds is common in children but may also be an indicator of an intestinal obstruction.

Abdominal pain in older children
Intestinal obstruction

This may have various causes. One is intussusception, which occurs usually between the ages of three and nine months. This is an infolding of a segment of bowel, causing obstruction that may need surgical repair. It affects previously healthy, well-nourished infants, coming on so suddenly that she may wake with a surprised shriek of pain. There are then inter-mittent attacks of severe cramps, sweating and dis-turbed sleep. Other symptoms are:

- vomiting of greenish-yellow material;
- failure to pass stools;
- later, passage of blood-stained mucus;
- fever and swelling of the abdomen if treatment is delayed.

The above symptoms require urgent attention. Call an ambulance.

Appendicitis

This is fairly common in children. The appendix, a worm-like structure attached to the large bowel in the right lower abdomen, easily becomes obstructed or infected. Symptoms appear fairly suddenly, with pain in the centre of the abdomen which steadily worsens, and later becomes localized in the right lower abdomen. Slight pressure on the tummy increases the pain. There is some nausea or vomiting, and fever. If neglected, the appendix can burst, resulting in an abscess or infection of the abdominal cavity – a very serious condition called acute peritonitis.

Acute abdominal pain in children may also be caused by inflamed glands in the abdomen (mesen-teric adenitis), secondary to a throat infection. This can be difficult to distinguish from appendicitis.

Position of the appendix

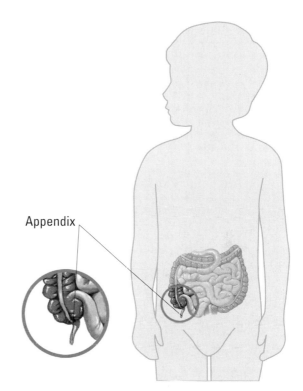

Appendix

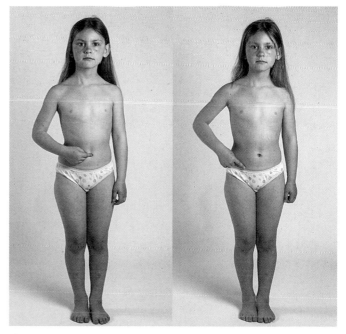

Appendicitis pain usually begins at the navel and moves down toward the right lower abdomen.

Another cause of acute abdominal pain is an infection of the bladder, tubes or kidneys (*see* Urinary Tract and Genital Problems, pages 129–130).

➕ **FIRST AID** If your child has sudden abdominal pain, it is difficult to tell whether this is a temporary upset or something more serious. Do not give him painkillers or other remedies that may mask a serious condition. Do not give him anything to eat or drink. A hot water bottle held against the tummy may provide some relief. If symptoms are severe, or continue for more than three hours, get medical help.

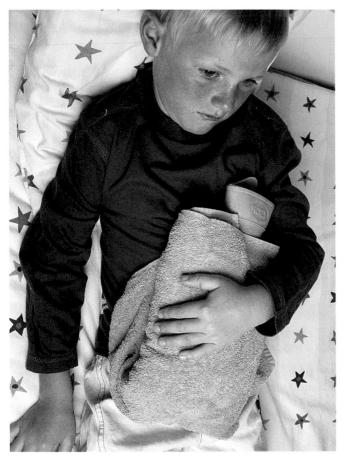

Place a hot water bottle – wrapped in a towel to prevent scalding – on the abdomen to relieve pain.

Functional abdominal pain

About 10–15% of children will experience recurrent abdominal pain, particularly if they are highly strung and anxious. It is rare before five years of age and is most frequent between 10 and 12. No cause for the pain can be found, so we term this 'functional' abdominal pain. The pain is generally vague and in the centre of the abdomen. It seldom wakes a child from sleep. If it does, you should suspect a more serious cause, particularly if the pain is not in the centre of the abdomen but to one side.

If your child has this kind of pain without any other symptoms, get him checked by a doctor to make sure there are no other possible causes. Your doctor will assure you that, although there is no serious illness, the pain is real and not in the child's head – which will help relieve your anxiety and the child's. The next step is to discover what is troubling him and deal with any stresses within the home, school or peer group. Abdominal pains of this kind should then become fewer and less frequent. It is not a good idea to give medicines to such children.

Some young children (one to five years) who experience attacks of abdominal pain at intervals of weeks or months, with or without vomiting, will later display the classic symptoms of migraine, especially if there is a family history of migraine (*see* Recurrent Headaches, page 117).

Constipation

Children differ in the frequency with which they pass stools. As long as the stools are soft and normal in consistency and are passed painlessly, do not worry about regularity. Constipation is the infrequent passage of hard stools with straining and discomfort. Although it may seem a minor problem, it can become a major one for an older child as a result of over-forceful toilet training as an infant, a painful anal fissure, or even reluctance to use unsanitary toilets at school.

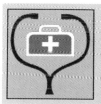 **FIRST AID** Constipation is rare in breast-fed babies, although stools may be passed only every five to seven days, but a baby fed on cow's milk formulae may pass hard stools. To relieve constipation in babies:

- add 2.5ml (half a teaspoon) of brown sugar to each feed;
- increase fluids by giving the baby more water or fruit juice during the day;
- give 5ml (one teaspoon) of prune juice as a laxative if the problem persists.

To relieve constipation in older children:

- see that they drink plenty of fluids;
- ensure they get roughage in their diet (cereal, brown bread, vegetables and fruit);
- get them into the habit of regular, unhurried toilet visits each morning.

Consult your doctor if your child's constipation does not improve, or the abdomen is painful or swollen.

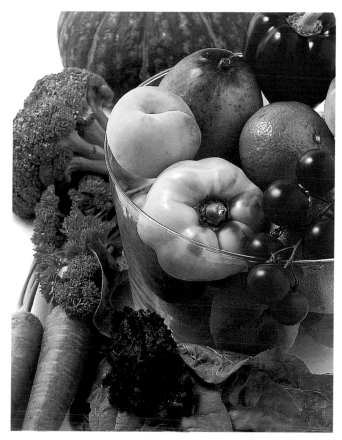

Fibre in vegetables and fruit helps to prevent constipation naturally.

Anal fissure

Sometimes a small tear in the lining of the anus may result when the child passes a large, hard stool. This causes pain on defaecation and the stool may show a streak of fresh blood. Treat this promptly.

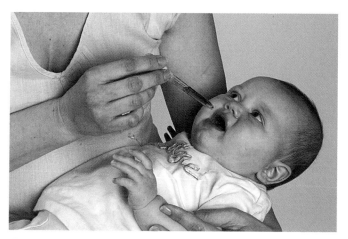

A teaspoon of prune juice can relieve persistent constipation problems in babies.

FIRST AID Buy a mild anaesthetic cream from your pharmacist (for example, Remicaine™) and apply it with your little finger, gently inserted into the anus. Repeat three times a day, and before a stool is passed.

Give the child a stool softener such as Dufalac™ for a week, or give a vegetable laxative (Senokot™) every night for one week.

Worms

Two common types of worms in the bowel are round-worms and thread (or pin) worms.

Roundworm

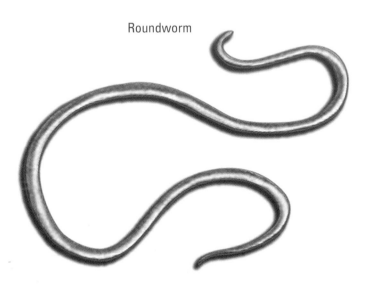

Roundworms

Roundworms are much larger than threadworms – up to 15cm (6in). One or two may be found in the child's stool, or may even be vomited up. When there are large numbers of worms in the bowel they can become knotted up and cause an obstruction. Occasionally worms get stuck in odd places – resulting, for example, in an obstructed appendix or bile duct. If the child has been infested with roundworms for a long time, larval worms passing through the lungs may cause persistent wheezing or pneumonia.

Other worms, such as hookworm, whipworm and tapeworm, are less common in temperate climates but can cause more severe symptoms.

Threadworms

Threadworms are tiny white worms that live in the lower bowel. The only symptoms are itching around the anus caused by the sticky eggs they deposit. There may be infection from the child's scratching. The worms may be seen wriggling in the stool. In girls the vulva may also be itchy.

Threadworms are easily spread from one child to another by eggs transferred on the fingers, so ensure you teach your children to wash their hands regularly, especially in daycare centres and wherever they use an outdoor play area. Also remember to make sure that you wash vegetables thoroughly.

✚ **FIRST AID** All worms are easily eliminated by modern medications (abendazole or mebendazole), which are safe and effective. Consult your pharmacist.

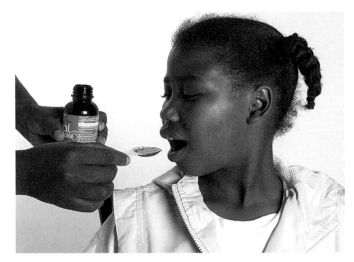

Intestinal worms can easily be eliminated with the appropriate medication.

URINARY TRACT AND GENITAL PROBLEMS

Urinary tract infections (UTIs) are infections of the bladder and the tubes carrying urine from the kidneys – the ureters and urethra. They are more common in girls, as the urethra is much shorter than in boys, so bacteria can more easily enter the bladder from the bowel.

URINARY TRACT INFECTIONS

Learn to recognize UTI symptoms, such as:

- burning on passing water;
- unusual frequency of passing water;
- bed wetting in a previously dry child;
- in children under two, diarrhoea;
- urine that is smoky or pink in colour and may be odd-smelling;
- fever, irritability and vomiting;
- pains in the back or abdomen (*see* Stomach Ailments and Abdominal Pain, pages 120–127).

Have a specimen of urine tested. Your doctor will explain how to collect it. If the doctor prescribes an antibiotic, make sure your child completes the course as prescribed.

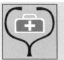 **See a doctor within 24 hours if you suspect a urinary tract infection.**

The urinary tract

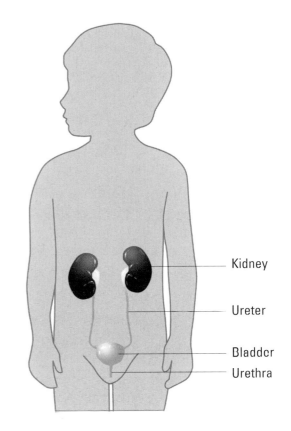

Kidney

Ureter

Bladder
Urethra

How can UTIs be prevented?

Children should be encouraged to pass urine every four hours or before each meal and especially before going to bed. It is a good idea to encourage 'double urination' in a child who has had a UTI – going back a second time and trying to produce a drop or two more. Both girls and boys should be encouraged to wipe their bottoms from front to back after using the toilet.

Girls' problems
Vulvovaginitis

Burning or itching of the vulval area, vaginal discharge and discomfort on passing water may be caused by:

- infrequent changing of nappies and poor hygiene;
- wearing tight pantyhose (tights);

- bubble baths;
- threadworm infestation;
- in older girls, thrush.

A smelly discharge may indicate a foreign body in the vagina (*see* Foreign Bodies in the Vagina, page 71).

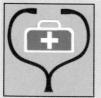 **FIRST AID** Sit her in a warm bath twice a day for a week, and wash her (or encourage her to wash herself) with a mild baby soap. Dry well and apply barrier cream, such as Siopel™ (see Nappy Rash, pages 135–136). Ensure she wears panties made of cotton rather than synthetic fabric, and she wipes herself from front to back after using the toilet.

If the problem persists, or symptoms are severe, consult your doctor.

Boys' problems
Balanitis
This is swelling and itching of the head of the penis and foreskin, with redness and a white discharge. As in vulvovaginitis, this usually results from poor hygiene.

 FIRST AID Wash the child (or encourage him to wash himself) regularly with a mild baby soap. Dry the area well and apply a barrier cream, such as Siopel™. Try to make sure he wears light cotton underwear rather than synthetic fabrics.

> **If the problem persists, or symptoms are severe, consult your doctor. Circumcision may be needed in severe cases.**

Phimosis
This means an unretractable foreskin, which is normal in infancy. In some boys the foreskin is not retractable till the age of four.

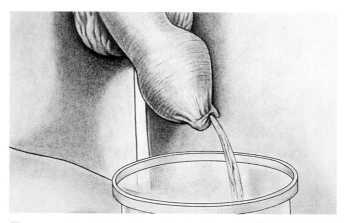

The opening in the foreskin is abnormally small in phimosis, which may make passing urine difficult.

Paraphimosis
This term means a retracted foreskin, which is stuck behind the glans, causing severe pain and swelling.

> **Seek medical help urgently.**

Torsion of the testis
The testis can become twisted on its appendages, causing severe pain. The scrotum on the affected side is swollen and red and the testis hard and extremely tender to touch. In an infant, the cause of the screaming may not be apparent until the genitalia are examined.

> **Seek medical help urgently. This condition requires immediate surgery.**

RASHES AND SPOTS

Your child has a rash...

This chapter describes some common childhood rashes. There are a number of other less common ones, some of them serious, some not. If your child develops a rash that does not fit any of these descriptions, see a doctor as soon as possible.

Many childhood infections cause rashes. They can be:
- spotty rashes (multiple pink spots, either flat or slightly raised);
- patchy rashes (irregularly shaped patches or generalized redness);
- blistery rashes;
- blood spots in the skin.

Most rashes are not serious, but some are outward signs of an infection needing urgent medical attention. Consult a doctor about any rash occurring with fever, in case it is measles, which is a serious illness. Any blistery rash in a very young infant requires urgent attention.

(For advice on general management of rashes with fever, *see* Fever, page 103, and Respiratory Tract and Lung Disorders, pages 104–106.)

SPOTTY RASHES

Probably the commonest rash in children under two is a virus infection called 'rose rash' (*roseola infantum*). It usually starts with three days of high fever and irritability, after which light pink spots appear on the body. The temperature then settles and the child feels better. There are no other symptoms, although there may occasionally be a febrile convulsion at the start, as the temperature rises very suddenly (*see* Convulsions and Seizures, pages 118–119). The condition is mostly harmless.

✚ FIRST AID You do not need to do anything other than bring the child's temperature down if he feels uncomfortable (*see* Fever, page 103). Give lots of fluids. Once the rash appears, the temperature will go down and the child will be well again.

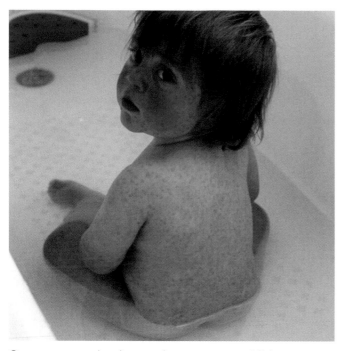

German measles is not dangerous to children.

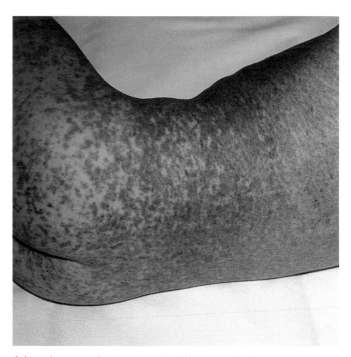

Measles can be prevented by vaccination.

German measles (rubella)

German measles is caused by the rubella virus and usually occurs in children over two who have not been vaccinated against it. There is very little fever. The child simply feels unwell and has a rash lasting for two or three days. At first the rash is separate pink spots, mostly on the trunk. On the second day it runs together into a generalized redness and then fades. The glands at the back of the head and in the neck are usually enlarged. Older children may have sore joints for some weeks after an attack of rubella.

✚ FIRST AID Unless the rash causes discomfort, you do not have to do anything. However, it is advisable to have a doctor confirm the diagnosis, because rubella is dangerous to a woman in the first three months of pregnancy. Her growing embryo can develop serious eye, ear, brain and heart problems.

Measles

This is the most serious of the common childhood rashes. It is extremely contagious, and is most severe in infants and in children who are weak or chronically ill. It is a notifiable disease. Thanks to an effective vaccine it is now uncommon but still accounts for 50% of deaths from common vaccine-preventable illnesses in poorer countries.

Measles starts with fever, cold symptoms and red eyes, all of which get steadily worse for four or five days before the rash appears. The child is sickest as the rash is coming out, which can take as long as three days. It starts as spots and blotches deep in the skin of the face, neck and chest. These spread to the rest of the body and the limbs. Because the virus also affects the lining of the respiratory and digestive tracts, cough and diarrhoea are common additional symptoms, and the illness may be complicated by ear infection, severe croup or pneumonia.

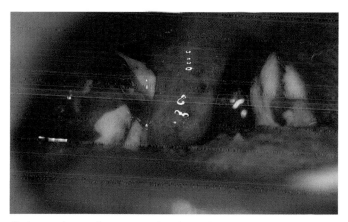

FIRST AID If your child is feverish, give paracetamol (acetaminophen) syrup eight-hourly as needed. Give plenty of fluids, and small, regular meals. A multivitamin mixture (especially with Vitamin A) will protect against secondary infections.

Ensure your baby is vaccinated against measles.

Glandular fever (infectious mononucleosis)

This is a common viral infection in older children. The symptoms usually include a sore throat and enlarged tonsils, as well as enlarged glands in the neck, armpits or groin. If it is incorrectly diagnosed as 'strep throat' and treated with an antibiotic, the child may develop a spotty rash.

Enlarged tonsils covered with white membranes (resembling strep throat) are characteristic of glandular fever.

FIRST AID There is no specific treatment for glandular fever, but the child is likely to be tired and listless for some weeks. See your doctor if you are worried. She can check him for possible complications, such as disorders of the blood or nervous system.

PATCHY RASHES
Scarlet fever

Now uncommon, scarlet fever is caused by a streptococcus, which produces a toxin that causes a red rash. It starts suddenly, with high fever, sore throat, headache and vomiting. Within 12 hours the rash appears, first on the neck and chest, then the rest of the body. The face is flushed, with a pale area around the mouth. Tonsils and throat are inflamed and the tongue is white-coated. After a few days the coating peels off, leaving a red tongue with redder taste buds (a 'strawberry tongue'). Skin affected by the rash feels rough. After a week there is peeling, especially of the palms and soles.

FIRST AID Consult a doctor to confirm the diagnosis. She will prescribe an antibiotic to shorten the course of the illness and prevent complications, such as rheumatic fever and kidney disease. Make sure your child takes the full course.

Give paracetamol (acetaminophen) liquid to reduce high fever and make the child more comfortable. Keep him away from other children for a week.

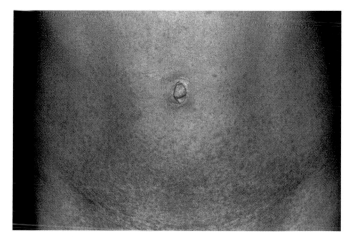

Scarlet fever – also known as scarlatina – produces a sore throat with widespread rash.

Slapped cheek disease

This common mild illness seldom has complications. It is caused by a virus that is widespread in the community, so young children are often infected without any symptoms. Typically, the child comes home from school with very red cheeks, as though he has been slapped. There are no other symptoms and no fever of note. A pink spotty rash then comes out on the trunk and spreads to the limbs, forming an irregular lacy or spotty appearance. The rash can persist on the limbs for as long as six weeks but the child remains quite well.

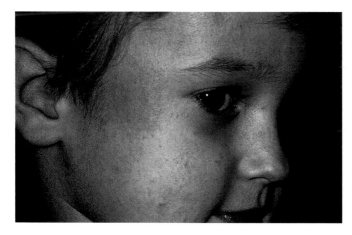

Slapped cheek disease is not accompanied by fever.

➕ **FIRST AID** No specific treatment is required, but keep the child away from any pregnant woman, because if she is not immune the foetus may be severely affected. The virus may also badly affect children with chronic illnesses.

BLISTERY RASHES
Chicken pox

This infection, caused by a virus, is generally a mild illness in children but more severe in older people. Typically there are only a few hours of fever and feeling unwell, then small red spots appear, usually on the trunk. These rapidly become small round blisters containing clear fluid. Soon more appear elsewhere and the process continues for a day or two. The severity of the rash varies, from only a few spots to involvement of the whole body. The blisters are itchy and easily popped on scratching. The resulting little ulcers turn into scabs and often become secondarily infected. Sometimes there are a few blisters inside the mouth and in the genital area. The scalp almost always has a blister or two – a good way of telling that the rash is chicken pox.

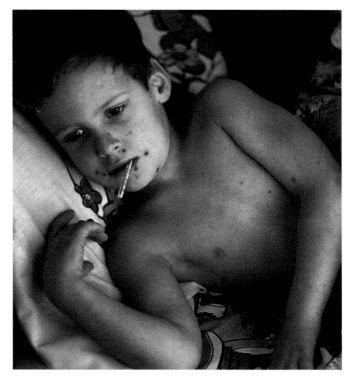

Small, round, red blisters containing clear fluid are characteristic of chicken pox.

➕ **FIRST AID** Apply calamine lotion to relieve itching and dry the sores. Consult a doctor, who may prescribe antibiotics for secondary infection of the blisters, and watch for any unusual complications.

Hand, foot and mouth disease

This viral infection causes blisters on the arms and legs, as well as mouth ulcers (*see* Hand, Foot and Mouth Disease, page 112).

Blood spots under the skin

You can tell a rash is caused by bleeding under the skin if the spots do not fade when you press them. These can be tiny bleeding spots or larger ones (bruises).

Bruises are usually caused by the mishaps that are a fact of life for all children. Sometimes small blood spots under the skin may be caused by the pressure of a garment, such as sleeping in clothing with a raised pattern, when the spots take on its pattern on the chest or abdomen. However, bleeding into and under the skin is a symptom of a number of significant, though generally rare, conditions so get a doctor's advice unless the cause is obvious.

Meningococcal infection

Meningococcus is a bacterium that causes a dangerous blood infection, sometimes also meningitis (*see* page 117).

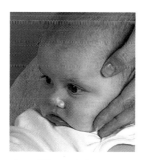

A stiff neck is a sign of meningitis.

The illness usually starts with fever and a few small blood spots that appear any-where on the body, including the eyes and mouth. There are often early signs of meningitis (headache, vomiting and stiff-ness of the neck). In the most severe cases there is widespread progressive bruising, shock and collapse.

See your doctor immediately if you see blood spots or bruises in your child's skin, unless you know they were caused by a bump or a fall.

Bleeding into the skin and elsewhere may follow viral illnesses such as rubella or chicken pox.

Seborrhoeic dermatitis

This is common in babies between one and six months. It generally gets better by itself. The baby may have thick greasy crusts (cradle cap) on the scalp, neck, nose and ears and red scaly patches on the body. The neck, groin and armpits may become reddened and weepy, which can lead to secondary infection by yeasts or bacteria. The rash does not itch, and causes little discomfort.

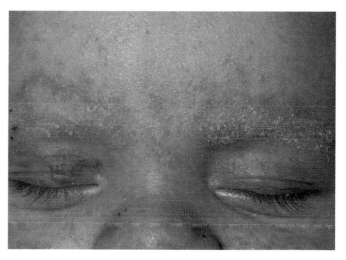

Greasy scales on eyebrows and forehead indicate that the baby has seborrhoeic dermatitis.

+ FIRST AID Remove the scales and crusts by massaging olive oil into the scalp and leaving it on overnight. Then shampoo and gently remove the scales with a comb. Regular bathing and short periods of exposure to sunlight are often beneficial.

Get medical advice if the rash is infected.

Nappy rash

A baby's skin easily becomes irritated or infected if he wears a soiled nappy for too long. There are many kinds of nappy (diaper) rash. At first all you may see is redness over the buttocks or thighs, around the anus,

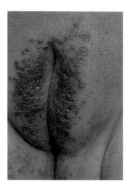

Raw skin and blisters make nappy rash a source of great discomfort.

or in the skin folds of the groin. Later the area becomes inflamed and weepy, and there may even be blisters or raw open areas. When there is a yeast (candida) infection you will see roundish red patches that spread and are scaly around the edges.

The main causes of nappy rash are heat, damp, friction and diarrhoea. Less commonly, it may be an allergy to elastic, soap powder or fabric softener.

➕ **FIRST AID** Change the nappy more often, cleaning the skin thoroughly each time with warm water and mild baby soap. Dry thoroughly and apply a protective cream such as zinc oxide ointment, Fissan Paste™, Nivea™, or a barrier cream such as Siopel™.

Good hygiene and short periods of exposure to sunlight will help prevent more severe rashes. For severe rash ask your pharmacist for an effective anti-bacterial, anti-fungal and anti-inflammatory cream. See your doctor if the rash does not clear up or if the baby is also unwell or not thriving.

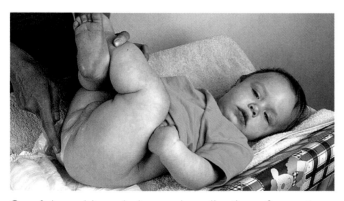

Careful washing, drying and application of a protective cream helps prevent nappy rash.

Impetigo

This is an infection caused by skin bacteria (staphylococcus or streptococcus). It appears as golden crusted sores or pus-filled blisters anywhere on the body. Staph infection is more likely if there are sores on the face, and if it started by itself, not with scratching. Strep impetigo tends to occur with scabies and insect bites, which the child scratches. It is found more often on the child's legs and produces more severe skin damage. If the lymph glands in the groin, armpits or elsewhere are enlarged, strep is more likely.

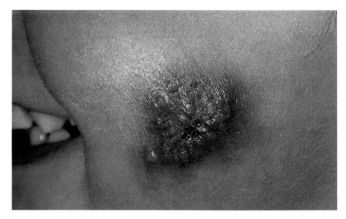

Impetigo sores are often covered by golden crusts.

➕ **FIRST AID** Consult your doctor for a prescription for the appropriate oral antibiotic treatment. Treat the rash with Vioform™ emulsion or povidine-iodine cream, but never with anti-histamine or antibiotic creams.

Boils

Boils are caused by the same germs as impetigo, but the infection starts off in a hair follicle rather than in the surface skin, producing a painful red swelling. The boil gradually comes to a head and discharges pus, bringing relief. It can occur anywhere on the body. A splinter or small wound may be the entry point for infection.

⊕ FIRST AID If the boil is small and not causing much pain, apply a poultice – a paste made of Epsom salts (magnesium sulphate) and a little warm water. Cover with gauze to encourage the boil to come to a head. When it bursts, gently wipe the pus away with cotton wool soaked in antiseptic. Cover it with a dressing, kept in place with pieces of plaster placed well away from the boil. Do not apply sticking plaster to the boil itself and never squeeze or poke the boil.

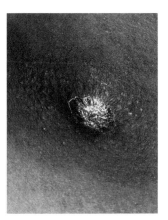

A boil is a round sore with a yellow head surrounded by tender redness.

A large boil that is very painful, or one that is getting bigger or not coming to a head after two days, must be opened by a doctor as soon as possible.

⊞ Get medical help if:

- the child has a fever or is unwell;
- the child has recurrent boils;
- you see red lines extending from the boil – this indicates a more serious condition (cellulitis) that requires urgent attention.

Recurrent boils

When boils occur recurrently on the head and neck, or on the buttocks and lower half of the body, your child may be harbouring a staphylococcus germ in the nose or anogenital region.

Sometimes recurrent boils are a sign of a more serious condition, so get a medical check-up to obtain the correct treatment.

Fingernail infections (whitlows)

A finger (less often, a toe) may become infected at the side of or under the nail. The side of the finger is red, tender and swollen, and a yellow head of pus may form.

⊕ FIRST AID Soak the finger for 15 minutes three times a day in warm water containing a little antiseptic. You can apply a poultice as for boils. If the whitlow comes to a head, you may be able to release the pus by gently pushing the skin aside at the edge of the nail.

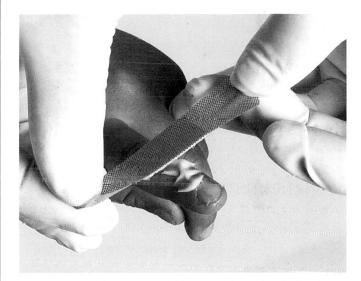

Apply a poultice to a whitlow to clear the infection.

⊞ See your doctor if:

- the finger is swollen and tender;
- the finger has not improved in 48 hours;
- the infection has not completely cleared within seven days.

Styes

These are boils that affect the eyelashes (*see* Styes, page 116).

Eczema

Eczema – like hay fever and asthma – commonly runs in families. Children with eczema are generally allergic to several things, though seldom to foodstuffs. The rash is intensely itchy, red and often weepy.

In young children the cheeks, forearms, front of the legs and trunk are most often affected. In older children the front of the elbows and back of the knees are more commonly involved, and the itchy skin is dry, cracked and often thickened.

➕ **FIRST AID** A child with eczema must see the doctor. The condition is treated by applying plenty of moisturizing creams, using topical cortico-steroids where necessary, and using wet wraps.

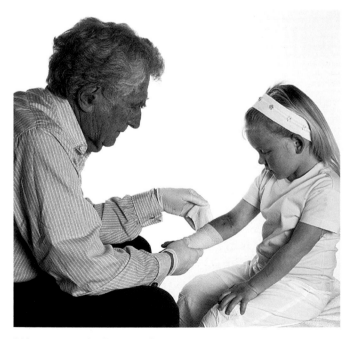

Wet wraps help to relieve eczema.

Wet wraps are cotton bandages moistened with hot water, applied to the affected areas and kept in place for up to 24 hours at a time. Apply them daily at first, and then less often as the skin heals. Stop when the itch-scratch-itch habit is controlled, but continue if the child starts to scratch again. This extremely effective treatment is recommended by dermatologists.

Some children develop chronic, non-itchy, pale patches, with a fine scale that looks like bran on the face or neck (*pityriasis sicca alba*). The cause is unknown, but it may be a mild form of eczema. Consult your doctor for appropriate medication.

A rash around a child's mouth may be due to the habit of lip-licking or lip-sucking ('lick eczema'). Moisturizing creams can help, or consult your doctor.

Psoriasis

This is a common chronic skin complaint that runs in families and is marked by sudden flare-ups with long remissions inbetween. It consists of red, scaly, thick-ened patches, which are not particularly itchy but may be uncomfortable, mostly on the scalp, elbows, knees and lower back.

➕ **FIRST AID** Control mild cases by keeping the skin well moisturized with aqueous cream and exposing affected areas to the sun for short periods.

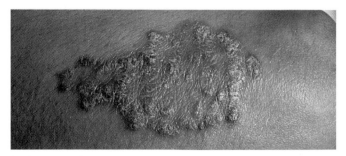

Raised, red, scaly patches are typical of psoriasis.

In more severe and distressing cases, consult a doctor, preferably a dermatologist, as there is a range of effective remedies she can recommend.

Urticaria (hives or nettle rash)
Urticaria may be caused by a virus infection or an allergic reaction to a foodstuff, drug or insect sting. It is an intensely itchy rash consisting of irregularly shaped, slightly raised pale blotches surrounded by a red border (weals). It may cover a small area or be very widespread. The weals shift their position – each one rarely lasts longer than 12 to 24 hours.

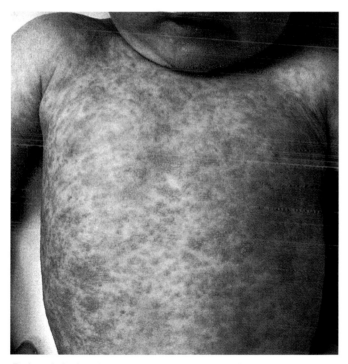

Raised, itchy, irregularly shaped patches are indications of urticaria.

⊕ FIRST AID Antihistamine syrup or tablets from your pharmacy may relieve the symptoms. If your child has chronic urticaria (recurring frequently or lasting longer than six weeks) see the doctor so the

cause can be identified and eliminated. In severe cases there may be facial swelling, even anaphylactic shock. An adrenaline injection under the skin is often effective (*see* Anaphylactic Shock, pages 107–108).

Pityriasis rosea
This starts as a ring-worm-like patch on the trunk, followed five days later by a rash on the trunk, but not the face. It consists of fawn-coloured or dark pink, slightly scaly spots that follow the lines of the ribs, so that they have a 'Christmas tree' distribution. Sometimes there is

The trunk is covered by slightly scaly patches that do not itch.

mild itching, but no other symptoms. It is a harmless condition of unknown cause that tends to occur seasonally and gets better by itself. Exposure to sunshine or ultraviolet lamp treatment helps it get better faster.

Warts
These are caused by a virus infection which may spread from one child to another. Common warts are raised, have a rough surface and usually affect the hands and feet. Plane warts are flatter, with a smooth surface, and affect the face, neck or hands. Warts are harmless

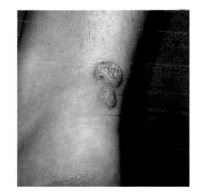

Warts are best left alone unless they are in an awkward spot.

growths which are best left alone as they generally disappear in six to 12 months. However, a wart on the sole of the foot (plantar wart) can be very painful and requires treatment. Otherwise, treat a wart if it is in an awkward place or if it looks ugly and your child is embarrassed about it.

FIRST AID Cover the wart with a wart plaster, and change it daily. For a plantar wart, first remove the layer of hard skin with a pumice stone before applying a plaster. Where a plaster cannot be applied, use a wart paint daily until the wart disappears, first protecting surrounding skin with petroleum jelly. Get plasters and paint from a pharmacy. If the child has many warts, a doctor can remove them with liquid nitrogen.

 See a doctor for warts on the face.

Another common childhood skin condition is *molluscum contagiosum* – pearly white or pink nodules, often with a dent in the centre, appearing on the trunk, face or hands. These are contagious and caused by a virus. They are best left alone, as they disappear in time, but see the doctor if the child has a large number of them.

FUNGAL INFECTIONS

Fungi are yeast-like organisms that are widespread in the environment. Some may cause skin problems. Children may get infected by touching animals, from contact with other children, their clothing, or the soil.

Ringworm of the body

This is a fungal infection of the non-hairy skin, the face being particularly affected in children. The circular or oval patches have a well-defined raised border and they gradually enlarge as they clear in the centre.

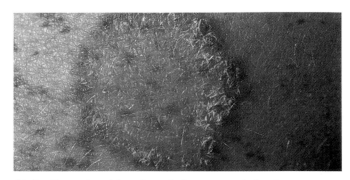

Note the raised border of ringworm infection.

FIRST AID Ringworm can be cured by applying anti-fungal skin cream daily for two to three weeks. Ask your pharmacist about suitable medication.

Ringworm of the scalp

Here the fungus establishes itself deep in the hair roots, making hairs break off close to the skin and leaving a large scaly bald patch or several smaller patches over the scalp. In the early stages it may resemble severe dandruff. If the child develops an allergy to the fungus, the patches become inflamed, weepy and crusted, and the glands at the back of the head and neck become enlarged.

Ringworm of the scalp can be confused with other conditions such as impetigo, so consult your doctor for diagnosis and treatment.

Pityriasis versicolor

This is a fungal disorder that causes multiple small patches with clearly defined borders. They may be lighter or darker than the surrounding skin. The upper portion of the trunk, neck and lower half of the face are most often affected.

FIRST AID Consult your doctor for a diagnosis and a prescription for a suitable anti-fungal treatment that you can apply at home.

Athlete's foot

This fungal infection cause itchiness and cracked tender skin between the toes. Toenails sometimes become thickened, discoloured and cracked. It is usually acquired from the floors of communal changing rooms and swimming baths. It is not common before puberty.

⊕ FIRST AID Effective remedies are available; ask your pharmacist to recommend one.

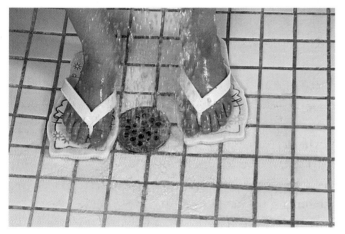

Use slip-on rubber sandals in public showers.

SCABIES

Extremely itchy, this is caused by sensitization to scabies mites, or their eggs and excreta. Mites burrow into the skin, preferring the chest, abdomen, genitalia and extremities, particularly wrists and hands. In hot climates they remain in the top skin layers, producing only small raised spots. In cold climates the burrows go deeper to form little lines. Children usually catch scabies from skin-to-skin contact, not from clothing and bed linen.

Suspect scabies if a rash is extremely itchy and friends or family members have it too. It is highly contagious so it is essential to treat the whole family. Consult your pharmacist.

⊕ FIRST AID An effective, safe, and cosmetically acceptable treatment is Permethrin™ (synthetic pyrethrin). Benzyl benzoate can also be used but is less pleasant. Other remedies are crotamiton, sulphur cream, and Tetmosol™ soap, but none will cure severe cases.

HEAD LICE

Lice are a common infestation of the scalp in children. The eggs (nits) can be seen as little white specks glued to the scalp hairs. The adult louse feeds on blood by biting into the scalp, producing itchy raised spots which often become infected from scratching, resulting in impetigo of the scalp. The lymph glands in the child's neck are frequently enlarged. As with scabies, treat the whole family, as the condition is highly contagious. Consult your pharmacist.

⊕ FIRST AID Permethrin™ scalp lotion is a safe and effective treatment. This kills nits as well as lice, so that the hair need not be cut or shaved. Malathion™ (0.5% in alcohol) or benzyl benzoate can also be used.

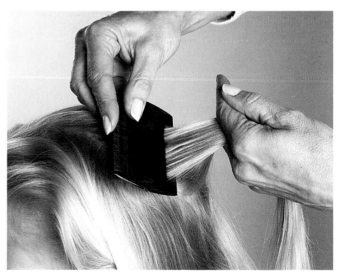

After shampooing, comb out nits with a lice comb.

IMMUNIZATION

Immunization is a simple, effective way of protecting children against dangerous illnesses. There are some infections the human body cannot make itself immune to without help. Give your child this help by seeing that she gets the right vaccines so her body will develop immunity. This also helps others, because if the level of immunity in the community is high enough, then the infection cannot spread so easily from one person to another.

IMMUNIZATION SCHEDULE

At birth	Polio and BCG
6 weeks	DPT, Polio, Hep B and HiB
10 weeks	DPT, Polio, Hep B and HiB
14 weeks	DPT, Polio, Hep B and HiB
9 months	Measles
18 months	Booster DPT, Polio, Measles or MMR
5 years	Booster DT, Polio, Measles or MMR

FREQUENTLY ASKED QUESTIONS
What do these abbreviations mean?

BCG is the Bacillus Calmette-Guérin vaccine, for protection against tuberculosis (TB).

DPT is the combined Diphtheria, Pertussis (whooping cough) and Tetanus vaccine.

DT is the Diphtheria and Tetanus vaccine, without Pertussis.

Hep B is the Hepatitis B vaccine.

HiB is the Haemophilus influenzae B vaccine.

Measles is the anti-measles vaccine.

MMR is the combined Measles-Mumps-Rubella vaccine.

Polio is the Poliomyelitis immunization – the injected Salk vaccine or the oral Sabin one.

Can I expect a reaction after immunization?

Mild fever and irritability are common, particularly after DPT, Measles and MMR immunizations. With DPT this occurs six to 12 hours after the injection. The site of the injection may also be red or sore for a day or two. With Measles and MMR, mild fever can be expected about seven days after vaccination. Some 10–20% of infants will develop a slight rash or other measles-like symptoms. There are virtually no reactions after the Hepatitis B and HiB vaccines.

Side-effects can be alleviated by giving three doses of paracetamol (acetaminophen) in the recommended dosage at four-hourly intervals. If a child has shown more severe reactions to a particular vaccine it should not be given again. Consult your doctor.

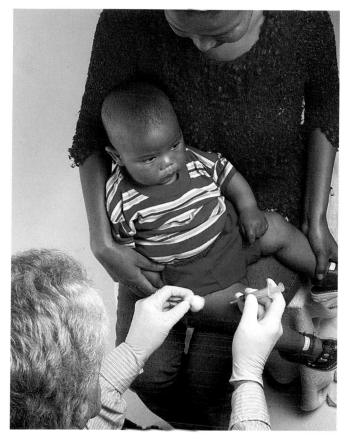

Immunization injections are not nice – but it is better to be safe than sorry.

My baby is allergic. Could immunizing him be dangerous?

If your child is allergic to something this does not mean he should not be immunized. Most of the genuine concerns are about the Measles and Mumps vaccines, as these are developed on chick embryos. The danger of an allergic reaction to egg protein in the vaccine has been exaggerated. Only if your child has shown severe allergy to egg, such as immediate swelling of the lips, difficulty with breathing, or a rash, should you avoid the Measles immunization. Very rarely a child may be allergic to the neomycin in the Measles vaccine or MMR, or to the carrying fluid in the DPT vaccine. If you are worried, consult your doctor.

Does immunization cause cot deaths or autism?

Extensive research has shown that immunization does not cause either of these conditions.

Can the Polio vaccine cause paralysis?

Most Western countries are using the Salk vaccine in which the virus is inactivated. With this vaccine there are virtually no reactions.

With the oral Sabin Polio vaccine there is a genuine, though extremely small, risk. This vaccine contains live altered viral particles which spread the immunity to polio around the community. As a result – although rarely – the child himself, or one of his contacts, is paralyzed by the virus, just as happens with real ('wild') polio.

In Africa and some other countries, the oral Sabin vaccine is still widely used because it is effective and cheap and spreads immunity through the community. As a result of its use polio has virtually been eliminated throughout the world.

My baby was premature. Is she too delicate to be immunized?

Premature infants respond to immunization just as well as mature babies and should be immunized at the same time intervals after delivery.

What about the child who is HIV positive?

These children are especially in need of protection. A child who is HIV positive should receive the regular schedule of immunizations.

Does my child really need the Hepatitis B vaccine?

Hepatitis B is endemic in less advantaged communities in many parts of the world. In these communities mothers can transmit the infection to their infants during or after pregnancy, or the children can acquire it later. But all individuals run a lifetime risk of becoming infected with Hepatitis B and should be protected. The vaccine is effective, cheap and very safe. All infants should receive it.

My neighbour's child has just been given 'H.flu' vaccine (HiB). Is it necessary?

Haemophilus influenzae type B (no relation to the influenza virus) causes severe infections in young children, particularly bacteraemia, meningitis and epiglottitis. The vaccine is effective and has virtually no side effects. All infants should receive it.

What about Mumps and Rubella?

MMR has been available for many years. It is very effective and safe, though expensive. In many countries it has replaced the single Measles vaccine.

What side effects can I expect in my baby after BCG vaccination?

This vaccination is given as a shallow injection into the skin of the right upper arm. A small pimple appears at the site, reaches its maximum size four to six weeks later, and may form a small scabbed sore. It gradually fades, leaving a scar. There is often an enlarged gland in the right armpit. These are normal reactions. Sometimes the sore on the arm may be bigger or the armpit gland may form an abscess. These reactions are generally not serious, but if you are worried, return to the clinic to have the baby assessed, or consult your doctor.

If BCG prevents tuberculosis, why is there still so much TB around?

No vaccine has yet been perfected to prevent tuberculosis. The BCG vaccine, in use for over 80 years, reduces the risk of some serious forms, such as tuberculous meningitis, found mostly in very young children. BCG does not prevent the tubercle bacillus from establishing itself in the lungs, so pulmonary TB remains common.

Is immunization permanent – or does it wear off?

The immunity conferred by the Pertussis (whooping cough) vaccine wears off, but the vaccine is not usually given after the age of 18 months because whooping cough is less dangerous to children after this age.

The immunity conferred by the Measles and the MMR vaccine may wear off in later childhood, so the child should get a booster when he starts school.

Although diphtheria is now almost unknown, Diphtheria vaccine boosters should be repeated every 10 years.

Immunity following the Polio vaccine is permanent.

The immunity conferred by the Tetanus vaccine does wear off, so a booster should be given if the child has a contaminated injury (see Tetanus, page 46).

Are there other vaccines my child should receive?

Consult your doctor about immunization not routinely given at clinics.

The flu vaccine is effective and safe and should be given annually to children with immune deficiency or any chronic illness. Such children should also receive the heptavalent (seven strain) pneumococcal vaccine to protect against serious pneumococcal infection.

A vaccine against chicken pox is available for children with certain disorders.

 Always consult your doctor if you are worried.

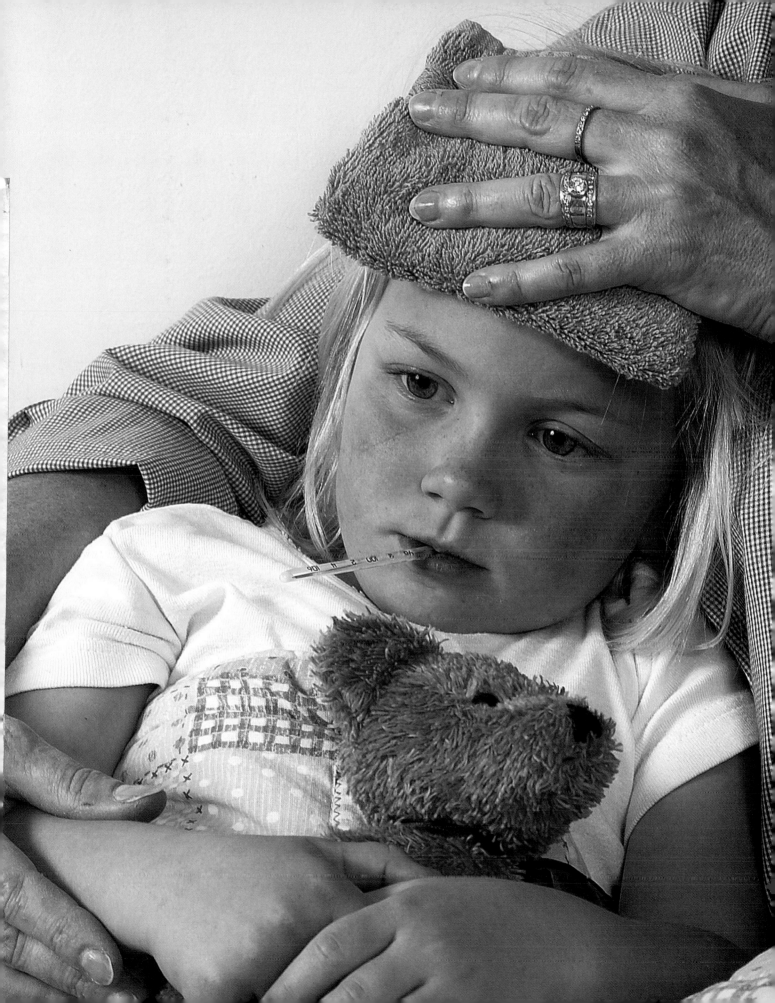

Acute Illness Table

✳ Go for it yourself

✳✳ Get a medical opinion (non-urgent)

✳✳✳ Get a medical opinion urgently

✳✳✳✳ Get medical help immediately

SYSTEM	DISORDER	SYMPTOMS	SEE PAGE	URGENCY
RESPIRATORY SYSTEM	Common cold	Watery nasal discharge, sneezing, cough, slight sore throat, maybe some fever	104	✳
	Influenza	High fever, headache, limb pains, cold symptoms	104	✳✳
	Sinusitis	Yellow nasal discharge, one or both sides. Pain over cheekbones or forehead; maybe swelling around one eye	105	✳✳
	Pharyngitis/ tonsillitis	Very painful, inflamed throat and/or tonsils, fever, enlarged tender glands below jaw angle	113	✳✳
	Nosebleeds	Bleeding from one or both nostrils; blood is often vomited up	114	✳ ✳✳✳ if it cannot be controlled
	Croup	Dry, barking cough, crowing sound on breathing in	108–109	✳✳✳

SYSTEM	DISORDER	SYMPTOMS	SEE PAGE	URGENCY
RESPIRATORY SYSTEM	Epiglottitis	High fever, malaise, difficulty breathing in and swallowing, loss of voice	109	✳✳✳✳
	Whooping cough (pertussis)	Cold and cough for one week; then regular spasms of coughing, ending in a whoop or vomiting, for up to three months	106	✳✳
	Bronchitis	Tight cough, 'phlegm on the chest' and wheezing on breathing out, usually following a cold; attacks are often recurrent	109	✳✳
	Asthma	Recurrent attacks of tight cough and wheezing, often at night or brought on by exercise; family history usually positive for asthma or other allergies	110	✳✳✳ full medical evaluation essential; then ✳ most attacks can be managed at home
	Anaphylactic shock	Increasing difficulty with breathing, shock and collapse, generalized itchy rash, swelling around the eyes.	107–108	✳✳✳✳
	Bronchiolitis	Infants under two years affected. Cold symptoms first; then slight fever, irritability, poor appetite, rapid shallow breathing	109–110	✳✳✳
	Pneumonia	High fever, cough, rapid breathing; may be chest or abdominal pain	106	✳✳✳ ✳✳✳✳ if danger signs (*see* page 106)

SYSTEM	DISORDER	SYMPTOMS	SEE PAGE	URGENCY
EYES AND EARS	Conjunctivitis	**Viral:** red eyes, irritation, watery discharge **Bacterial:** yellow discharge; eyelids matted together after sleeping Also caused by chemical irritation or allergy; both eyes almost always affected	115	✳✳ ✳✳✳ if only one eye affected, or if vision is affected, or cornea is abnormal
	Stye	Red, painful spot on eyelid which may discharge pus	116	✳ ✳✳ if recurrent
	Otitis media	Pain in one or both ears, hearing loss, maybe fever		✳✳ ✳✳✳ if severe pain
	Ear discharge	**Watery, mucoid** or **purulent (discharging pus):** ruptured drum following otitis media **Recurrent, purulent:** chronic perforation of drum **Bad smelling, purulent:** foreign body or mastoid (the hard area behind the ear) infection **Both ears, itchy:** external otitis	113–114	✳✳ ✳✳ ✳✳✳ ✳✳

SYSTEM	DISORDER	SYMPTOMS	SEE PAGE	URGENCY
NERVOUS SYSTEM	Meningitis	Headache, vomiting, stiff neck; listlessness, fever, maybe purple/red-brown spots on the skin	117	****
	Fits	Temporary disturbance of consciousness with or without stiffening or jerking.	116–117	***
DIGESTIVE SYSTEM	Oral thrush (candidiasis)	White patches on the tongue, inside cheeks or in throat; cannot be rubbed off without causing bleeding	111	* ** if persistent
	Gastroenteritis	Frequent loose stools, vomiting, abdominal cramps, may be some fever	121–123	* or **, depending on severity
	Dysentery	Frequent mucoid or blood-streaked stools, cramps and generally fever	121	***
	Intestinal obstruction	Bouts of central abdominal pain; vomiting bile; may be abdominal distension; no stools passed	124–125	***
	Pyloric stenosis	Recurring forceful vomiting 15 minutes after feeds, in infants one to four months old; weight loss and constipation		***
	Intussusception	Sudden onset of bouts of severe abdominal pain in infants under two years; constipated, but may pass blood-stained mucus ('redcurrant jelly')	125	****

SYSTEM	DISORDER	SYMPTOMS	SEE PAGE	URGENCY
DIGESTIVE SYSTEM	Acute appendicitis	Central abdominal pain and vomiting, pain then localizes to right lower abdomen, which is tender to pressure; may be some fever	125–126	✳✳✳✳
	Mesenteric adenitis	Central abdominal pain, fever, may be sore throat	125	✳✳✳
	Hernias: 1. Inguinal/groin (strangulated)	A lump in the groin which does not disappear on gentle pressure; maybe symptoms of intestinal obstruction as above	124	✳✳✳✳
	2. Umbilical	Swelling at the umbilicus caused by bowel herniating through a weak spot; seldom obstructs	124	✳✳
	Anal fissure	Painful passage of hard motion streaked with blood	127	✳
	Acute hepatitis	Loss of appetite, malaise, some fever; upper abdominal pain and tenderness; then urine becomes dark brown in colour; yellowness of skin		✳✳
	Worm infestation: 1. Roundworms	Worms in stool or worm is vomited	128	✳
	2. Thread (pin) worms	Anal itching	128	✳
	3. Whipworms	May cause mucoid, bloody stools	128	✳✳
	4. Hookworm	Anaemia	128	✳✳
	5. Tapeworm	Segments in stool	128	✳

SYSTEM	DISORDER	SYMPTOMS	SEE PAGE	URGENCY
URINARY TRACT AND GENITALIA	Urinary tract infection	General symptoms: fever, irritability, vomiting, diarrhoea (children under two years) In older children: frequency and burning on passing water; pains in back or abdomen, bed wetting (when previously dry); urine smoky or pink, maybe odd-smelling	129	✲✲
	Glomerulo-nephritis	Urine brown, reddish or smoky, output diminished; Swelling around the eyes, later more generalized; may be headache		✲✲
	Vulvovaginitis	Burning or itching of vulval area; vaginal discharge; discomfort on passing water	129–130	✲ ✲✲ if severe, or if molestation a possibility
	Torsion of testis	Tender tense swelling high in the scrotum	130	✲✲✲✲
	Balanitis	Swelling, itching of head of penis and foreskin, redness and white discharge	130	✲✲
	Paraphimosis	Retracted foreskin, cannot be replaced	130	✲✲ ✲✲✲ if over four years
	Phimosis	Unretractable foreskin	130	✲

SYSTEM	DISORDER	SYMPTOMS	SEE PAGE	URGENCY
MUSCLES, BONES AND JOINTS	Arthritis	Pain on movement of one or more joints; may be swelling of joint(s)		✻ ✻ ✻
	Osteomyelitis	Fever, pain, maybe swelling and redness of affected limb		✻ ✻ ✻
BLOOD DISORDERS	Anaemia	Unusual paleness of palms of hands; also of tongue, lips, eyes (conjunctivae)		✻ ✻
	Purpura	Tiny bleeding spots in skin or mucous membranes; unduly easy or spontaneous bruising or bleeding		✻ ✻ ✻ ✻
LYMPH NODES (GLANDS)	Enlarged lymph nodes	Small painless nodes (under 1cm) may be felt in healthy children in neck, below angle of jaw, in groin		✻ ✻ ✻ if nodes are tender, suddenly appear, or any node is larger than 1cm
INFECTIOUS DISEASES	Roseola	High fever, irritability for three days; then faint rash appears on trunk as fever subsides	131	✻ ✻
	Rubella	Slight fever, tiredness for a day, then spots appear	132	✻ ✻
	Measles	Fever, flu symptoms, maybe diarrhoea for three to five days, then rash	132–133	✻ ✻ ✻
	Scarlet fever	Fever, sore throat, headache, diffuse red rash on trunk	133	✻ ✻ ✻

SYSTEM	DISORDER	SYMPTOMS	SEE PAGE	URGENCY
INFECTIOUS DISEASES	Slapped cheek disease	Maybe slight fever and tiredness; red cheeks followed by rash on trunk; then lacy rash on limbs	134	✳✳
	Infectious mononucleosis	Inflamed throat, enlarged glands in neck, armpits, groins, may be spotty rash on trunk	133	✳✳
	Varicella	Crops of small blisters evolving into sores and scabs mostly on trunk; also in hair, in mouth, throat		✳✳
	Shingles (*herpes zoster*)	Crop of blisters on one side of head or body, ending at midline; usually not painful in children		✳✳
	Hand, foot and mouth disease	Small sores in the mouth or throat, followed by blisters symmetrically on hands, knees, feet	112	✳✳
	Herpetic stomatitis	Fever, sore throat, painful sores in mouth; red, swollen gums		✳✳
	Kawasaki disease	High prolonged fever; variable rash localizing to hands and feet; red lips and eyes		✳✳✳
	Tick bite fever	Fever, generalized papular rash, including palms and soles; tick bite	92	✳✳✳
	Mumps	Fever variable; swelling in front and below one or both ears or under chin	112	✳✳

SYSTEM	DISORDER	SYMPTOMS	SEE PAGE	URGENCY
SKIN DISORDERS	Nappy rash	Variable rash in nappy area	135–136	✳ ✳✳ if severe or infant not thriving
	Cradle cap	Greasy, yellow crusts or scales on scalp; red, scaly patches on trunk	135	✳
	Impetigo	Large blisters developing into golden crusted scabs	136	✳✳
	Cellulitis	Spreading area of redness, swelling and tenderness, often related to a break in the skin		✳✳✳
	Boil, carbuncle, stye	Painful papule developing pus at its head	136–137, 116	✳✳
	Scalded skin syndrome	Widespread blistering with loss of skin		✳✳✳✳
	Toxic shock syndrome	High fever, shock, maybe disturbed consciousness or respiratory difficulty		✳✳✳✳
	Urticaria	Irregularly shaped itchy papules which come and go; may be other signs of allergy	139	✳✳✳
	Papular urticaria	Fixed itchy papules, usually on legs and trunk	93	✳
	Warts	Firm raised growths with rough or smooth surface on hands, feet, face or elsewhere	139	✳ ✳✳ if multiple or on awkward spots

SYSTEM	DISORDER	SYMPTOMS	SEE PAGE	URGENCY
SKIN DISORDERS	Molluscum contagiosum	Pearly, dome-shaped nodules, often with central depression	154	✳ ✳✳ if multiple, or on eyelids
	Scabies	Tiny very itchy papules or small lines– wrists, between fingers, armpits, sides of trunk, genitalia; may be sores and scabs from scratching	141	✳✳
	Lice	Itching and tiny red spots on scalp; nits (small white eggs) attached to scalp hairs; lice may not be seen	141	✳
	Ringworm: 1. Of scalp	Early: general scaliness (like dandruff); OR round patch of hair loss with scaly surface; OR multiple bald scaly patches; OR multiple crusted lesions with enlarged neck glands	140	✳✳
	2. Of body	Scaly, round or irregular patch with clear-cut, slightly raised edge	140	✳
	Athlete's foot	Cracked skin with itching and soreness between toes	141	✳ ✳✳ if no improvement when treated
	Pityriasis rosea	Patch like ringworm on body; then multiple oval spots, slightly scaly, appear on trunk, lasting up to two months	139	✳✳
	Pityriasis versicolor	Discoloured patches of skin, slightly scaly, usually on neck and shoulders	140	✳✳

Glossary

Adenoids – Lymphatic tissue at back of upper throat

Anaesthetic (general) – Use of injected or inhaled drugs to induce unconsciousness for surgery

Anaesthetic (local) – Use of drugs to induce numbness in a specific area of the body for painless surgery

Anaphylaxis – Very severe form of allergic response, usually to foods, drugs, venomous bites or stings

Anti-histamine – Medication used to treat mild allergic disorders or reduce itching or skin irritation

Antiseptic – Prevents invasion or multiplication of bacteria, in order to reduce the risk of infection

Appendix – Worm-like attachment to the bowel in lower right abdomen

Artery – Blood vessel carrying blood from heart to organs

Asphyxiation *see* choking

Asthma – Condition causing recurrent wheezing, cough and breathing difficulty

Bacteraemia – Germs multiplying in the bloodstream

Bronchiolitis – Inflammation of the smallest tubes in the lungs

Bronchitis – Inflammation of larger branches of the airways coming off the trachea

Cardiac arrest – Cessation of normal heart beat; usually fatal

Cervical spine – portion of spinal column located in the neck

Choking – Inability to breathe due to obstruction in the upper airway

Chronic infection – Infection that persists despite treatment, or recurs intermittently over period of time

Circulation – Collective term describing the blood, heart and blood vessels

Clean – Free of any dirt, and thus unlikely to harbour organisms which could cause infection

Compound fracture – Bone injury with associated damage to the neighbouring soft tissues

Conjunctivitis – Inflammation of the lining membrane of eye

Convulsions – Involuntary contraction of muscles caused by head injury, poisoning, or sometimes no obvious cause, as in epilepsy

Croup – Inflammation of upper airway, resulting in harsh cough and difficulty breathing in

Cystic fibrosis – Hereditary condition resulting in thick mucus

Dehydration – State whereby the body loses more fluid than is being replaced, with risk of damage to the brain or kidneys

Diarrhoea – Loose, frequent bowel motions

Dysentery – Infection in the large bowel, with loose stool containing blood and mucus

Epiglottitis – Inflammation of tissues just above the voice box

Gangrene – Irreversible destruction of tissue, most commonly as a result of poor circulation

Gastroenteritis – Bowel infection causing vomiting and/or diarrhoea

Haematoma (bruise) – Collection of blood caused by a damaged blood vessel

Haemorrhage – Significant loss of blood from any part of the body

Hernia – Rupture

Immunization – Artificially induced protection against certain illnesses **Laryngitis** – Inflammation of the voice box

Ligaments – Tough groups of fibres, usually attaching bones

Lymph glands – Small fleshy glands, mostly located in neck, groin and armpit; can become swollen and enlarged as a result of infection

Meningitis – Inflammation of the membranes around the brain

Migraine – Recurrent headaches, often with nausea and/or vomiting

Mumps – Viral infection causing swelling of the salivary glands

Otitis media – Inflammation in the cavity behind the eardrum

Papular (rash) – Describes skin rashes where the markings are red and raised above the normal skin surface, e.g. papular urticaria

Peritonitis – Inflammation of inner lining of abdomen

Pertussis – Whooping cough

Plaster of Paris – White, powdery substance, usually coating bandages used to make nerve impulses from most parts of the body; enclosed and protected by the vertebral column (backbone)

Sterile – Free of any bacteria or other organisms

Suffocation – Inability to obtain enough oxygen due to lack of oxygen in the atmosphere, or obstruction of the mouth and nose

Supine (position) – Lying on the back, facing upward

Systemic (generalized) – Term describing any symptom or condition involving the entire body rather than just one area

Testis – Testicle; the male semen-secreting gland

Tonsils – Pair of lymphatic organs at entrance to throat

Tourniquet – Any material that encircles a limb tightly, and may obstruct the blood supply to the rest of the limb (we do not recommend its use)

Trachea – Main tube through which air passes to and from lungs (windpipe)

Vaccination *see* immunization

Wheezing – Breathing difficulty resulting in whistling sound on breathing out